UNDOING BANDAGES: A PLASTIC NOVEL

Sylvester Fernandes

Ruby Press

For more information, or to book an event, contact :
Email :info@svfernandes.com.au
Website http:www.svfernandes.com
ISBN - Paperback: 978-0-6458543-0-5
ISBN - ebook : 978-0-6458543-1-2

First Edition: July 2023

Dedicated to the memory of my mother, Petolina, my father, Desiderio and my sister, Senhorina and all the giants who have allowed me to stand on their shoulders.

1

The plane taxied the tarmac metamorphosing the recently sprayed lavender fragrance in the cabin into human sweat smells and then ascended as if it was in a great hurry at Heathrow Airport in London towards the stratosphere. James' thoughts alighted to the recent job which he was now vacating in Leeds. The plane had its usual quota of homeward bound, attention detracting Indians to contend with and threaten his accumulating thoughts. This Indian platoon would have shamed the biblical tower of Babel with their cacophony except somehow they seemed to understand each other as manifested by the grinning and pendulous side to side neck movements. It was obvious that they would not have actually cooperated voluntarily in a joint venture involving the construction of a tower and particularly if any biblical connotations were involved. To escape the ennui some of the other passengers had resorted to snoring loudly, as their contribution to the prevailing din.

Although currently sardined in his seat, Dr. James Regan usually projected precisely five feet seven inches from the ground and like his name sake, *James Dean* had a triangular face with the vertex subjected to a greater gravitational force and a dimple plastered onto the chin. He had deep set blue eyes that seemed to have a question for any viewers in his direction. His nose appeared to ski towards his philtrum and in no apparent hurry. His hair was light brown and sinuous as if to impede the audiowaves above his head and cause them to undergo a phase shift. He was twenty nine years old and had just finished his Senior Registrar training in Leeds, and was more than glad to escape the cold English snow clad weather and burrow back to his hometown, Newcastle, Australia where he had secured an appointment as a plastic surgeon at the Royal Newcastle Hospital, where he had trained earlier in his career.

Reflecting on his experiences in the last two years as a senior registrar in Leeds, he reminisced that life had been pretty mundane apart from the busy clinics and the heavily booked National Health Service outpatient sessions and the operating lists that allowed for nothing else apart from restricted and minimal daily living activities and some failed romantic encounters mainly due to his unencumbered intolerance of the Yorkshire ritual incantations of "yes luv" and "coop of tea" that incensed his entire being, and his uncompromising preferences of female superficial anatomy.

He remembered some funny episodes which usually haunt the memories of most doctors, contributed to by fellow doctors and patients.

He remembered the incident when a paediatric patient for the revision of a birthmark on her face proposed to him.

"Will you marry me? I cook like mum."

"When?" he inquired to keep her attention going.

"Tomorrow after Sunday," was her honest reply.

She was immediately silenced by her mother with threats of post consultation ice cream deprivation, putting an end to the marriage proposal which incidentally may have been his first.

He was also reminded of the sycophant female patient who had travelled from Riyadh expecting a cosmetic rhinoplasty done free of charge, under the National Health Scheme and when disappointed to learn that such was not possible, had immediately produced a huge wad of British currency notes and pushed it into his hands in the outpatient department, much to his embarrassment. How the nurses had all gathered around him with amazing alacrity to protect their colonial buddy! She then showered some language constrained vituperative abuse decipherable only by the tempo and tone of her voice, into James' face, aided by the movement of her right index finger. Such inconveniences he hoped were now in the past.

The essentially heuristic clinical experiences at the Royal Leeds Hospital had been fruitful and he felt well prepared to meet almost any challenge that he might encounter in his future clinical practice. He also remembered how many long hours he had spent in the hospital library equipping himself to go ahead with an impending operation he had not done before and with no consultant supervision available, he was on his own. Nevertheless he had benefitted from these solo experiences which had significantly improved his confidence. He particularly felt most confident in lip and cleft palate surgery which he was planning to subspecialise in. However he would need to do general plastic surgery initially for a while, whilst he established his presence in Newcastle. As he reminisced, he was joyed that soon he would be able to plan his own schedule undictated by other circumstances. Or so he preferred to think now and decided to turn his attention to his immediate surroundings.

On his left near the window was a young Indian woman bedecked with gold ornamentation, to include nose, ear and several digit and wrist rings and was appropriately labelled with a red dot on her forehead and with a perpetually fixated smile that she imparted on all objects, animate and inanimate in her visible vicinity. The smile may have been an attempt by her to blend in with the prevailing sentient and insentient milieu without hurting any feelings, possibly an aftermath of her ingrained beliefs. She was claiming her own territory in the plane with coconut oil pheromones.

On the aisle side was an Indian gentleman who threatened the seams of his coat with his every movement, to include even his own breathing. James saw the man's presence there as a warning to keep his own fluid intake low as it may cause a massive disruption to the prevailing equilibrium which had just been established with several intonations of pain, and implorations to several deities of the *hare khrisna* variety. And thus, his own use of the toilet would have to be restricted. His seat was also being submerged under instruction from the gentleman's overflowing adiposity. How lucky it was that the gentleman occupied the aisle seat! He only hoped the Indian woman on the window side would also be cooperative in this particular matter.

"What can I get you sir?" inquired the friendly airline hostess as she met James' gaze.

"Just a neat scotch whiskey would be great. Thank you," he responded.

"No problem."

The whiskey arrived a few minutes later along with the requests from his neighbours for just plain water.

As he was savouring his drink, he pictured his mother, Elena and his dad, Rodney and Janet, his sister waiting for him at Kingsford Smith Airport in Sydney when his plane got there and then, the usual drive to Newcastle in his father's Jaguar 4.2 Sovereign, his position in the front passenger seat, and his mother and Janet in the back seat possibly listening to *Engelbert Humperdinck's* incantations or the baritone *Tom Jones*. If Elena had her way it would be *Kenny Rogers*. The Jaguar was a good car and had served the family well to date. When he could afford it, he may also buy a similar one, he thought.

His father, from whom he had inherited the gelasin on his chin, was an ear nose and throat surgeon at The Royal Newcastle Hospital. James was aware that his father was planning to retire in the next few years from clinical work, on to his vineyard estate and concentrate on cultivating shiraz grapes at Pokolbin in the Hunter Valley. To that end his father had done the requisite vigneron courses at the TAFE institute and also equipped himself with the requisite extra knowledge by associating on weekends with the local winemakers who were always helpful and ready to expose their experience by requesting his consumption of a bottle or two of their own wine as testimony. This usually terminated with Rodney buying a few bottles from the winemaker as expected, for home usage.

The Royal Newcastle Hospital was located with the Tasman Sea in the South Pacific Ocean on the rear and the city of Newcastle on the other. The views of the Ocean always haunted his memory during his time in England, when as a resident doctor there, a swim in the ocean in between the duties at the hospital was compulsively mandatory. Often romance aspiring nurses would join in. The oranges and sunshine days lie ahead again. Goodbye England. Nice knowing you. I will keep in touch. But now, I can hardly wait for the touch down at Sydney!

The whiskey had taken effect and he succumbed to the long awaiting sleep.
He woke up to find the plane had landed in Bombay

and was disgorging some passengers with the expected turmoil. After a while some newer ones arrived with similar vocal amplitudes and frequency characteristics to the disembarked ones to reinstate the Babel chaos scenario again.

Both the passengers on either side of him were gone and two Indian ladies both in jeans descended on the vacated seats. The one on the aisle side had the look of being released recently from a hostage situation and seemed to be on the lookout for more intrusion from her recent captors. She possibly surmised that James may be a member of the IRA or the like. One never knows, she thought. She vigorously avoided his visual interaction.

The lady on the window side smiled at James and looked for conversation.

"Hello my name is Guyatri. I am computer scientist and I work in Melbourne presently."

"I am James. I am a surgeon," James replied as he rolled his tongue.

The lady perceived that there may be some hidden meaning in his tongue rolling but was entirely clueless. What is the message he is trying to convey to me? Is he gluttonising over my breasts? Is he impressed that I am a computer scientist? She looked at him very closely searching for a meaning to his tongue rolling.

She did not want to miss any opportunity if it was knocking.

"Why are you going to Australia?" she inquired.

"I live there."

"Where?"

This inquisition was not to go on lightly James had guessed

"Newcastle."

"What were you doing in Bombay?"

"I came from London on this flight."

"Did your parents actually migrate or….."

James knew what this meant and was keen to escape the conversation. But how? He could go to the toilet. But the hostage woman would get more paranoid with this move as she was watching the toilet very closely. To have a terrorist sitting next to her would provoke in her, a greater anxiety.

"My great grandparents came from Ireland."

"Potato famine?"

"No, my great grandfather eloped to Australia with his cousin's wife."

This was not the answer she had wanted to receive and she immediately turned her face away expressing her nonapproval of his great grandfather's action.

He understood that Indians can be very judgemental and will often expect you to atone for the sins of your ancestors, a quality they share with Christian beliefs in crucifying Jesus for the sins of Adam and Eve. Indian inquisitions can be also be very prolonged with detailed attention to minutiae. He knew this from his stay in the United Kingdom and his encounters with the migrant Indian doctors there.

Perhaps this answer was subconsciously fortuitous. Peace will reign now, he hoped and it did.

On arrival at Kingsford Smith Airport, after the usual formalities of immigration and customs clearance were adhered to, James was able to locate his family in the waiting crowd. After the customary hugs and kisses, "You have lost weight James," Elena remarked.

"He's okay," Rodney said.

Janet was just looking at him and smiling. It was obvious she was delighted to have him back.

"I will get the car around," Rodney volunteered at last.

The sky outside was blue and cloud deprived. A few added clouds and it could be a *John Constable* painting about Suffolk, England. It reminded him of the National Gallery. He had been there a few times. He had also crossed the English Channel to visit the Louvre in Paris and it's very hyped *Mona Lisa*. He also did visit the Prada to appreciate *Diego Velázquez* particularly his *Las Meninas* which he loved and the Reina Sofia in Madrid which housed the *Guernica*. He remembered how he had spent a significant amount of time with the latter and had decided that he was really not fussed on cubism. He remembered how in school he was completely blown by a print version of Édouard Manet's, *A Bar at the Folies-Bergère*. He had seen it again at The Courtaurd Gallery on the Strand in London and virtually did not sleep that night. Art did have a profound effect on him. He thought about the miserable weather there in Europe to ease his pain. He was going to miss all that art here but heck, this is home!

Apart from his love of art, James had other qualities of note. He had an immense hunger for knowledge and could and would spend any available hours in reading. His memory was very impressive and he could remember minute details of topics he had read several years ago. And as if this was not enough, his choice of subjects was very varied and ranged from ant warfare to elephant skin grafting. His only worry to date was - there was so much more to know and so little time!

And there were things he hated. Most of all he did not like people who indulged in 'small talk'.

The drive home in the Jaguar was smooth as could be expected. There was not much changed in the scenery outside. Some new estates with houses under varying stages of construction lie on either side. Otherwise the drive was materially uneventful.

"How did you cope with the weather in England?" Elena asked.

"Very well. I loved the spring and autumn most. The spring season is beautiful. All the lovely daffodils particularly in the Lake District."

"I have to get there one day," Janet said.

"Autumn, with all the falling leaves," James continued.

"Yes its beautiful isn't it?" Rodney remembered.

"Almost makes you sit down and write poetry," James continued.

"The ideal place for poets. In fact the land of poets, *William Wordsworth*, *John Drinkwater* come to mind," Rodney remembered.

"Winter and snow and Christmas is quite exciting at first, but after a while it drags you down," James continued.

"I could never be bored by snow," Janet remarked.

"Tell me about the food," Elena wanted to know.

"The Indian food is great. *Rogan josh curry, Tandoori chicken.*"

"What do the English mainly eat?" Elena continued.

"Fish and chips," James replied.

"Not meat pies like us?" Janet questioned.

"Did you meet Lord Heartley on Harley Street?" Rodney asked.

"No. I rang his rooms once. They said he was on a lecture tour in the US and won't be back for three months. I did not try again," James replied.

"We both passed the fellowship exam together," Rodney was keen to inform.

"Maybe you should visit him one day," James advised.

"I have thought about that. But I don't think my arthritis would appreciate that weather now."

"Jamie if you go back, I'm coming with you," Janet said.

"I don't think he is in a hurry to go back soon darling," Elena interjected.

When they arrived at the Warners Bay house, James observed that the lawn was struggling to remain extant, "The lawn could do with some water."

"We have not been able to water the lawn for some time due to the restrictions," Elena explained.

"It will catch up in time," Rodney finished.

"The poms look after their tiny yards very well," James said.

"Tiny is exactly the right word," Rodney laughed.

"It's nice to see the little old ladies with white hair pottering about in the yard with their teacups and cutting the beautifully coloured flowers. They appear to be in constant conversation with the plants. I am sure that's all they do the whole day apart from consuming their cups of tea."

"I will help Jamie with the bags. You girls go in. We will both have a whiskey when we come in. You can join us if you wish," Rodney offered.

On entering James could smell the sandalwood candles that Janet preferred in the house. She had done an evening course in aroma therapy and then decided the sandal wood was best for enhancing the mood and sensual feelings. Rodney and Elena had not noticed any benefits so far. The general décor in the house had not changed. The velvet red sofas still fought for the available space and it appeared that the hardly ever used fireplace had already found its grave. As a child James could remember how his mother was reluctant to use the fireplace as it taxed her cleaning prowess.

The crystal chandelier with its shiny wide range of colours which commanded James' prolonged attention as a child was still welcoming.

"How does it feel to be home?" Janet inquired.

"Really great Mercury," James replied.

"You have not changed. Or maybe we are still seeing the same side of you again," Janet remarked.

He knew he was home and amongst his own kin.

Tomorrow he had to be at the hospital outpatient department. He hoped he would be able to cope on the first day and not be bothered by too much jetlag. He wondered what it would be like to get back at the Royal and which of his old residency colleagues would still be there?

2

James was keen to get moving on the next day and set his feet into the hospital. He drove in early and parked his car at one of the unmarked spaces. The disinfectant smell was strong. He sauntered along the corridors of the hospital trying to look both important and knowledgeable, towards the out patients section where his initial encounter was programmed. A senior nurse recognised him on the way, "Doctor Regan how nice to see you back."

"I'm glad to be back too, Emma" he breathed in his familiarity rolling his tongue.

"You are looking well. How long have you been away. It seems like only yesterday."

"About two years."

"Where did you go?"

"England."

"How nice. I want to go there sometime."

"You must. The poms are nice people."

"I'm sure they are. Except that I haven't met the nice ones yet. Perhaps the nice ones stay at home to look after their mothers. But more of that later. I will catch up with you later in outpatients," and she hurried off.

"Sure, see you then," he rolled his tongue.

He walked away contented that in his absence in the last two years he was not entirely forgotten and resumed his saunter.

The outpatient department was located in the old building and was easily locatable by the ambient din of the mothers small chatting and the crying children who would prefer to be anywhere else.

"What's wrong with your child?" one mother inquired of another.

"He has a testicle mark which the family doctor wanted me to check out," and the minimal vestments of the child were removed to expose the anomaly, and as evidence for the statement.

"Mine has a lip problem. He finds it difficult to suck."

"That must be hard. How do you manage?"

"The nurse showed me how to hold him and the bottle. We have nipples with several holes. We manage."

"I suppose he will need surgery"

"Yes. I am told Dr. Regan specialises in this kind of surgery"

The nurses had their own contributions to make to the prevailing din, employing raised voices to gain the attention of the waiting patients, and also to express their frustration and anger. The patients and their accompanying relations were assembled in chairs which were vacated in sequence as the queue progressed to see the doctor.

The plastic surgery section was shared with the ear nose throat and also the dental surgeons on different days of the week. James' occupancy was delegated for Tuesdays. He had two co–plastic surgeons, Drs Eleanor McEwen and Damien White in the department with their own separate units who used the out patients on other days.

James had a registrar and a senior and a junior resident in his unit. A passing intern attempting to fulfil mandatory requirements for medical registration was always available for the senior doctors to vent their frustrations. The prime duty of the intern was to do as told and not to reason why.

James and the registrar, Matt and the residents Pete and Mohan occupied separate rooms in the outpatient department. The intern sat in with James to watch and wrote the requisite forms for clinical tests or operating theatre bookings. James insisted that the intern be with him. He felt it best that the intern could make the better decisions for his career if he learned straight from the horse's mouth! The residents consulted the registrar for cases that challenged their knowledge or how to proceed and the registrar consulted James under similar circumstances.

When James found an interesting teaching case, the registrar and the residents were summoned to his room and their ignorance explored politely.

And so now they assembled in James' room at James' request.

"This 38 year old gentleman is a boilermaker at BHP Limited and complains of increasing right wrist pain of at least six months duration. He relates it to a fall about one year ago. Initially the pain was localised but now there is stiffness, clicking and grinding and crescendo pain with motion," James began.

The registrar compared both hands and noted there was pain on pressure in the right wrist. He also noted that there was some swelling and motion was painful.

"What to do next?" James rolled his tongue.

"Xray," the junior resident volunteered

James produced the xrays and put them on the viewing box.

"The lunate bone appears dense," the registrar screwed his eyes at the box.

"Yes, correct, so?" James pushed further for a response..

"Post traumatic arthritis," the registrar replied.

"What else? We need differentials,"James continued

"Rheumatoid, fractures," the registrar attempted.

"What about *Kienbock*?"

"Could be," the registrar who was due for the second part of the fellowship exam agreed.

"Do you guys know what Kienbocks disease is?" James asked the residents. "Perhaps you can tell them about it later," James motioned to the registrar. "And whilst you are at it don't forget to revise the anastomosis around the wrist. The examiners love to ask that question if you ever get this case"

The registrar and residents left nodding their assent.

James felt good he had found an interesting case for the juniors today to expose some of his knowledge. He remembered that he saw a similar case in England which ultimately ended in fusion surgery.

A while later, the registrar came into James' room requesting his attention with a case of left mandibular branch facial paralysis following facelift surgery about two months ago. The patient was a forty plus woman. The registrar wanted to know if facial nerve grafting could be considered.

After James examined the patient and the investigations, "I think that cross facial nerve grafting could be considered. Perhaps Damien may be interested. You might want to ask him."

"Okay," and the registrar walked out with the patient.

A bit later, Pete the resident requested his attention on a case.

"This is Mr Alistair Thomson. He is thirty-seven years old and is a mine worker. He has this brown nodule on his back which has enlarged in the last month. He says it is itchy and often bleeds. I think it warrants an excision biopsy. No axillary nodes are palpable. Can I put him on tomorrow's list?"

"Yes definitely. It looks like a melanoma to me"

The other outpatients provided no real challenges to James today. There were the usual burn scars which required grafting. A diabetic with *Dupuytren's* contractures of the hand and another with alcohol concerns also commanded his attention. An adolescent girl with a post injury nose deformity requiring rhinoplasty was also drafted for further surgical attention. He felt he had enough work to last a comfortable operating session. There were more patients waiting on his lists currently, left by previous occupants of the position to last at least for another four weeks.

"That's it for you Dr Regan" the nurse came in to inform him.

"Okay. Have the others finished?"

"No. The have a few more patients"

"In that case I will wait till they are finished. I could do with a coop of tea whilst I am waiting"

"You will need to get rid of your Midlands accent here. This is Australia. Nevertheless I will get you a coop," and she smiled.

"Just testing."

The residents and registrar assembled in James' room after they finished.

"Guys this is my first day on the job. How did I go?"

"Feedback time huh," the registrar smiled.

"Yes. We can all learn."

I wish I could tell him to stop his tongue gymnastics, the intern thought. It is so very irritating. I wonder if he is married. Who could put up with that? But lucky I am not here to stay.

To gain their confidence James inquired," What are you planning to do Pete?"

"Ear nose and throat, if I can."

"That's a cut throat business," James laughed, appreciating his own pun. "And you Mohan?"

"Neurosurgery."

"That's good."

The intern watched the floor awaiting his turn, if any. He was contemplating and prioritising the calls he had to attend to when this compulsory episode in his life was over.

"What about you Brad? Have you made up your mind yet?"

"I am leaning toward general practice at present."

"You have no intentions of specialising?"

"I thought about psychiatry. I did a term there and I

was convinced it was not for me."

"Ah well, each to his own."

"Matt, is there anyone you want me to see in the wards?"

"Not today."

"By the way before I forget, before you put anybody on the operating list, always seek clearance from me."

"That's a given." Matt reassured

James was mentally fatigued for the day and on that note they parted.

On the way to his Mazda, James' memories raced back to the days when he was a young intern, not very confident of himself but was mostly never bullied by his seniors as the other juniors usually were and he knew it was due to his paternal intangible leverage in the hospital.

He met Damien, his co surgeon on the way, "Hello Damien, how are you?"

"I am well James. Good to see you back. When did you get back?"

"Yesterday. I still feel a bit pooped."

"I am sure you do. You are too keen James, as usual. You have not changed. What else have you being doing extracurricular?"

"The British system keeps you very busy. Not much time for anything else. What about you?"

"As it was in the beginning."

"Are you married yet?"

"Yes. I got married last year. I don't think know her. She is a school friend of my sister and is now her sister in law"

"Interesting. I presume your romantic pursuit has been long and purposeful. Where do you live?"

"New Lambton. You must come over one day when you are less pooped."

"Yes I will. Incidentally my sergeant, registrar I mean. You know Matt. Matt has an interesting case for you for possible cross facial nerve grafting. He will be in touch with you soon."

"Sure, I will look forward to that," Damien retorted but wished his true thoughts could be known. Do I really need that? I have enough cases of my own. Please pretend I do not exist in future.

"I'm glad. Okay, I will see you later." James sought his leave. As he walked away James felt lucky he had such collaborative company.

"Yeah. See you." Damien walked away briskly not wanting to look back as if he did not wish to be burdened with any more cases.

On his way home James was pleased that his first day had gone well. No hiccups at all. Tomorrow, operating start at 8.00 am. Must remember to set the alarm. Must also look around for an apartment to stay. Close to the hospital. But perhaps not. Maybe three bedrooms.

When he got home Elena opened the door.

"Jamie is home" she announced.

Rodney was also at home parked on a sofa and guiding some whiskey into his mouth.

"How was your first day?" Rodney inquired.

"Very good. No problems. I have some nice residents."

"Good."

"I met Damien on the way out."

"Damien White?"

"Yes, my co-surgeon."

"He doesn't like to work. I think he would prefer a more sinecure job."

"Really?" James realised his earlier error but he was not able to correct it now.

"Pour yourself a whiskey and join me."

"That I shall do," and he went off to find the whiskey and poured himself a large one.

Elena busied herself finding some nuts and crisps.

"Mum would you like a drink?" James asked.

"Yes, Some Bombay gin and tonic Jamie. Thanks."

When they were seated the dog came in and settled at Rodney's feet ensuring him a fall if required.

"What time is Janet coming home?" James inquired.

"Not too late I hope. I must tell you about this interesting book that I read," Elena continued.

"What was it about?" James wanted to know.

"Bullshit." Elena completed.

"Was that the title or the contents?" Rodney was interested.

"I picked it up at the second hand bookshop for two dollars. It is called *On Bullshit* by *Harry Frankfurt*."

"Sounds interesting"

"He starts by saying that one of the most salient features of our culture is that there is so much bullshit. He distinguishes between lying and bullshitting."

"Which is?" James wanted to know.

"The liar and the bullshitter both try to get away with something. But 'lying' is perceived to be a conscious act of deception, whereas 'bullshitting is unconnected to a concern for truth."

"Almost everyone bullshits. Special commendations must go to our politicians and clerics," Rodney observed.

"According to Frankfurt, bullshit is unavoidable when people are convinced that they must have opinions about events and conditions in all parts of the world, about more or less anything and everything – so they speak quite extensively about things they know virtually nothing about," Elena explained.

"But eventually is there an objective truth? If there is, than truth has become less important than the demands of today's political, commercial, artistic and even scientific success," James added.

"Good point Jamie," Rodney complimented.

"You must read the book. Best two dollars I have spent for a long time"

"In fact *Rene Descartes* in his *Meditations on First Philosophy*, was struck by the large number of falsehoods that he had accepted as true in his childhood, and by the highly doubtful nature of the whole edifice that he had subsequently based on them that he summed up in *"cogito ergo sum*," Rodney provided

"We must be grateful for men like that. They have freed our minds," James added

"As I have always told you James, if you don't drive your Rolls Royce someone else will drive it for you," Rodney added

"Haven't got a Rolls Royce yet."

"I meant you mind. Regarding the real Rolls Royce its just a matter of time. The wait before consuming the marshmallows James."

"Got ya. The Stanford experiment."

At this point the doorbell rang and Janet arrived in.

She nodded to dad, "Hi Dad and all"

Rodney nodded back.

"Hello Mercury. How are you and what will you drink?" James inquired.

"Mum looks happy. I'll have what she is having, moon."

"Gin and tonic."

"Okay that's fine. Excuse me. I'll be back in a second."

All was quiet till Janet arrived back.

"Guess what? Mrs Armstrong aka Mrs strong arm wants me to teach physics next year and I am not happy," Janet began.

"Why? You have almost six months notice," Elena encouraged.

"Physics is the most basic of all subjects," James added.

"Mathematics is," Rodney replied.

"No. Mathematics was only invented to explain the discoveries of physics," James continued.

"I stand corrected," Rodney apologised.

"We had an interesting argument," James informed.

"About what?

"Bullshit," Elena replied.

"So what's new in this house?"

"No, we actually talked about why there is so much bullshit in this world and not much truth," James explained.

"The most effective bullshitters know the truth, including when to bullshit and when to give the straight shit. Even the school children are trained early," Janet explained her experiences.

"Bullshit really results from the adoption of stupid methods of justification, whether intentionally, blamelessly or as a result of self deception," Elena explained.

"The bullshitter knows very well what matters more than anything else to the person, just like the advertising industry exploits us," Janet added.

"We should be intellectually rigorous and detachedly rational if possible. Easier said than done, I will admit. Any bullshit that concerns our lives; our beliefs and certainties, including the ones that characterise our deepest convictions about ourselves and our ability to tell truth from falsity must be resisted. The more you know, the less bullshit you can tolerate."

"But sometimes it is difficult to tell the bullshitter off politely," Janet complained.

"I have a technique that I have developed over the years. Tune off. Watch but don't listen. Think of something else. Sometimes they get the message. I often use it at medical meetings."

"I need to do that more often," James confided.

"I want to read that book Lena. It sounds interesting," Rodney said.

"Me too," James said.

"I will go and fix dinner. I expect you all in the diner in fifteen minutes," Elena excused herself.

James was still in limbo about locating his private practice. He had much work to do on that front and several options to consider. He needed time to consider and did not wish to bother his dad at this stage.

3

James had decided that this was going to be an *annus mirabilis* and so far it appeared to be in gear.

He had marched down Bolton Street several times in anticipation of finding a place to set up his practice and noted the real estate availability around. Most of the medical consultants occupied the terraced houses toward the upper hilly end of the street towards the police station. His father Rodney had rooms located there and had offered to accommodate him initially till he could decide on a more permanent location. Parking on the street with the zoning restrictions was a nightmare. The wardens were always on the lookout for offenders who could help their own keep and their children's education and holidays. In general it was a situation where the educated employed funded the unemployed and unemployable, law abiding and law non abiding denizens of the city of Newcastle. It was obvious that he would have to rent a place in a car park, several metres away and walk the distance, meeting and greeting his patients along the way.

Learning from his own experiences and as per the demands of filial obligations, Rodney had informed him that the real estate agents and the car dealers were all behaviourally genetically derived from piranhas and leeches.

Shonie Alder, a long haired redhead, and Miriam Grey, longhaired and blonde, both excellent typists whom he knew from his residency days were recruited as his secretaries, along with nurse Jane Ponting, again a blonde who usually wore her hair in a bun and had worked with him in the past in the plastic surgery department at the hospital. All of them had several years experience and James was pleased with his choices.

He sent the requisite new private practice announcement letters and decided he would go around meeting referring doctors, some of whom were his co-residents, when he worked at the hospital. These practitioners were spread all around to include Newcastle, Lake Macquarie, Maitland and Cessnock.

In the suburb of Hamilton he went along to meet Dr. Ethan Whitehead, a co-resident with him in the bygone days, at the hospital. Dr. Whitehead was about his age and a well respected general practitioner in the locality now.

On introducing himself at the reception desk, the secretary asked him to take a seat.

The secretary went in to check Dr. Whitehead's availability.

"Doctor will see you now," the secretary came back.

James walked into the consulting room to see Dr. Whitehead already standing and extending him a handshake, "James, you are back .How good to see you."

"It's nice to see you too Ethan. You are looking very prosperous. Is that Porsche outside yours?"

"No, technically it belongs to my wife. But she allows me to use it all the time. She only sits on the driver's side and gives instructions."

"Let me guess. Mabel?"

"Mabel, it is. We get on well most of the time."

"So what is Mabel doing apart from putting up with you?"

"She gave up nursing and took up interior decorating. She is doing okay."

"I will need her services soon. Does she decorate surgeries?"

"She will help you with space allocation and choice of paint colours and things like that. You should come over for dinner one night and talk to her. She will be pleased to see you. Are you attached yet?"

"No."

"So you did not find a suitable in England either?"

"No.I could not stand the Yorkshire accent. I don't think I could put up with it for life."

"You have a point. For now, leave your phone number with my secretary at the desk. I will ring you this evening around seven. Is that okay?"

"Yes. That should be fine. I shall let you get on with the mob waiting outside. See you later."

"See you."

James left his telephone number at the reception desk and left. He was welcomed by the fiery sun that was waiting patiently outside for him. As he looked up toward the sky, he burst into a severe bout of sneezing. He hurried to his car to set off further in his Jamesian plastic surgeon proselytization mission.

On his way to see another one time co-resident who was now a general practitioner at Mayfield, James saw a surgery in Islington. He decided to drop in. A brass plate exposed the occupant doctor as Dr.Jagdish Jethani MBBS. He went in and introduced himself at the reception. He was immediately escorted in to the doctor after the elderly man who was being attended to, was requested to wait outside.

Dr Jethani wore a grey suit and had a weighty moustache that dragged his nose downward exposing a heavy growth of nose hair which danced with his breathing rhythm.

"Hello Dr. Jethani. My name is James Regan. I am a plastic surgeon starting practice in Newcastle," he uttered as he rolled his tongue.

"I am most pleased to meet you. It was very kind of you to drop in. We need more plastic surgeons here. It is hard to get appointments."

"I am available."

"Would you like a cup of tea? We have very nice Ceylon tea. Would you like some?"

For fear of being impolite and risking the consequences, James replied, "That would be nice."

Dr. Jethani called for his secretary and ordered her to make the tea.

"Make some tea for gentleman and me also."

In the interim James positioned him on his qualifications and experience.

"I have nephew in Bradford. He has Indian restaurant there."

"I have been to Bradford several times for medical meetings."

"Did you meet Kishore my nephew?"

"I don't think I have."

"You would know if you meet him. He is very nice man."

James was wishing the tea would arrive soon so he could escape this verbal biryani.

The tea arrived and James thanked the secretary as she left.

"I myself worked in the Royal Hospital personally about seven years ago for about three years in medicine branches," Dr Jethani volunteered.

"I don't it has changed much," James responded.

James gulped down the hot tea and was ready to leave.

"That was very good tea. You must excuse me. I have a lot of things to do today"

"You and your good wife must come over for a meal at my house in Lambton."

"Sure we will work something out," James was out of the door.

It was expected to be a perfect day outside according to the weather reports except it was not perfect .The sun had reached its highest meridian and the hot tea had exacerbated its effects. Nevertheless he was pleased that he had met Dr.Jethani although he was not happy to share an evening with him possibly devoid of alcohol imbibition, a vegetarian menu and the associated *vedic* wisdom. He will deal with the invitation when it arrives although he could plan his excuses in the meantime, he thought. To his delight the invitation never came but patients from Dr. Jethani did. It is often difficult to predict the referring doctors James learnt.

Ignoring the heat outside, he was on his way. His hospital colleague in the resident days, Dr.Peter Meaney was located in the Mayfield shopping centre with a pharmacist next door. James remembered Peter as always obliging and hoped he had not changed. He went in and introduced himself at the reception desk and was immediately ushered in.

Dr.Peter Meaney was a tall lean man who appeared to be perpetually on a fast and could do with some fat-laced food.

"James my friend, how nice to know you are back. How was England? Sit down."

"Very good and very cold."

"I just came back last week from my honeymoon from Fiji. Nice and warm there."

"Anybody I know?"

"I don't think so. She is a school friend of my sister."

"So she was a clandestine relationship that was not disclosed to us. You shifty mean Meaney."

"What about you? Are you hitched up yet?"

"No. Still looking."

"Ah well. Just a matter of time."

"I just dropped in to tell you I am starting my practice at Bolton Street with my father initially and then I will move out later."

"Well, leave your card in front and I shall see what I can do."

"Okay. Bye. I will catch up with you soon," and with that James lifted himself out of the chair.

"Yeah we should meet soon"

He left his card at the reception desk before leaving.

As he was leaving he felt happy. With friends like

these he should be okay in his practice. It took him some time to realise that all is not well that ends well. Dr Meaney never ever sent him any patients.

That evening Dr. Ethan Whitehead rang and invited him to dinner the following evening at his home in Merewether.

James arrived the next evening with a bottle of sauvignon blanc and flowers. The door was opened by Mabel who hugged him on seeing him.

"Mabel sweetheart, I shall never forgive you for choosing Ethan over me. You have wrecked my life forever."

"You have not changed one bit Jamesy. You must have left a few trusting broken hearts in England, hopefully, not pregnant."

"Okay, let's save the flattery and falsities for the politicians. Come in and sit down. What drink do you want to start with James?" Ethan interrupted.

"Here, I have some flowers for you Mabel. And what's left over can be yours Ethan." He handed the flowers to Mabel and the bottle to Ethan.

"You have not answered my question James?"

"I will have a whiskey with ice like old times."

"Yeah. You have not changed one bit as Mabel said. You will have the usual gin and tonic Mabel?" Ethan prodded on.

Mabel nodded and Ethan went off to fetch the drinks.

Mabel asked him to help himself to the nuts and soy and potato crisps which were prelaid in serving bowls on the coffee table.

Elvis Presley was admitting he was *All shook up* in the background.

The seating was mainly around the fireplace with an intervening coffee table. The fireplace was on vacation. The mantelpiece was of a minimalist décor with some decorated candle holders, a white abstract thinker figurine and their wedding portraits to justify their cohabitation. Hanging above the fireplace was a large picture of *Elvis Presley* exhibiting his erotic leg movements. Some books relating to interior decorating were lying on the buff wool pile carpet.

Ethan arrived with the drinks and after the usual "cheers" they inquired of James about his time in England. When that topic was exhausted, the current daily mundanity reigned in.

Mabel excused herself to set the table.

"I'll get you boys to reminisce old times at the Royal Hospital." She left for the kitchen.

"Thanks Mabel," Ethan responded.

"The good old times," James fashioned a smile.

"Yeah," Ethan chose his best smile.

"Hey do remember the time when Jason's parents arrived from Melbourne and we had Samantha walk out of his room nude? You should have seen the look on his mother's face. Jason never forgave me for that," James started.

"That was hilarious," Ethan laughed heartily.

"I wonder what happened to Samantha?"

"She is practising in Geelong. She married Louie the fly. She rings me sometimes."

"That marriage would be a mutual

misunderstanding   Say hi to them for me next time."

"What about the times you tried to fob off that waitress from the Seaberg Hotel? Remember the time she waited for you for six hours and you hid in Celia's toilet all the time and Celia had to use our toilet? I'm sure she had an inkling you were in there but she could not ask to inspect Celia's apartment, could she?" Ethan reminded him.

"Yes that was a death defying act going from our apartment to hers from the outside, with not many things to cling on to. Still sends shivers down my spine," James remembered.

"How stupid we were," Ethan admitted.

"Dinner is ready. We have chicken schnitzel and pavlova for desert," Mabel announced to the reminiscers.

"That's great," James replied.

Ethan poured some chardonnay in the glasses and another round of "cheers" followed. The meal continued with further reminiscences of the Royal until it was time to go, for James.

"It was good to see you James after all this time. Take care driving," Mabel farewelled.

"Yeah" Ethan repeated.

"Thank you for the evening," James replied as he left.

"*Show me the way to go home. I'm tired and I want to go bed...*" James sang as he went to his car.

The progress of establishing a private practice was relatively swift thanks to the astute guidance from Rodney who was aware of the swings and roundabouts of such from his own experience. Rodney introduced him to his own accountant and lawyer who were delighted to advise at special medical surcharge rates.

"Their fees are exorbitant aren't they," James was thinking about his National Health Service salaries.

"Ours are too," Rodney reminded James.

"So live and let live."

"Exactly."

He set up his rooms with his father. After an initial slow start the patients began to roll in. The appointment and operating lists were threatening to get out of control. Time seemed to be passing fast. There was usually no time for any amorous activity.

One late afternoon after he had seen his quota of patients, James stopped at the reception, "Hi girls, all going well?"

"Yes mostly" Shonie responded.

"Gosh you dad was really cranky with Ira Bunting today," Myrtle, one of his dad's secretary interfered.

"Ira Bunting who wanted a face lift?" James inquired.

"Yes That one."

"What about?"

"You know she has been a patient of your dad for several years. He complained that she always comes in with the same symptoms. This time what set him up was the collection of tissues she came with, appropriately dated and labelled. The tissues contained mucus from her left and right nostrils that she wanted him to see and feel. Oh how he complained! He said he was glad to retire soon just to regain his sanity."

"Well I'm glad I am not her bowel surgeon" James laughed which was echoed by them all.

As he was walking to the car he heard someone calling him from behind. He looked back and recognised Simon Schultz an old school friend who was teleologically ordained to sell insurance. He had sold his first instalment to James, when James was a resident. He was reminded of Simon's puerility in school particularly when one day Simon stole some viagra medication from his father's pharmacy and spiked the lunch of the school priests. It was funny to watch the priests going around as if they had unlighted torches under their soutanes. No one knew what exactly happened at that time and the priests were too embarrassed to open the matter up and no one was admonished. It was only a few years later, after they had left school that Simon told James about his role in the incident.

"Your girls told me you had just left and I may be able to catch you on your way to the car."

"It's good to see you Simon. What's up?"

"We have a new type of life insurance policy that you may be interested in."

"What, something that lays a bet on me lasting next year? I say, I will die. You say, no. I live. You win and get to keep the money. At the end of the year we bet again and you keep winning till I die."

Simon realised this may not be a good day to secure his custom.

"I will let you go James. I will catch up with you another time."

"Bye."

At home Rodney was already helping the whiskey to find a new rent free home in his gullet and James joined him.

"I heard you had a nasal secretory episode with Ira Bunting"

"She's a fruit cake."

"Don't tell me," James added

"I have never lost my temper with any patient but she brought me close today. I would have felt ashamed later and I'm glad I didn't. I just felt sorry for her."

"There was a surgeon I worked with in England, Mr David Shaw. He used to say some patients have an inborn rottweiler heritage. Once they bite a disease, they just don't let go," James said.

"I often see that with patients with a unilateral hearing loss. Some of them are convinced they have a tumour in their heads in spite of negative imaging."

"I can understand that," James said.

"They move from doctor to doctor till someone tells them that that there is indeed a tumour. That's the word they want to hear. This tumour, it's in your mind. This finally sets their mind at rest. All they wanted to hear is, the word tumour. Some of them do not know the difference between brain and mind. They go around promulgating, 'I always knew there was something wrong with me. Those other doctors were useless. All they did was collect the money.' These patients are now convinced and spread the news around how good their new doctor is until, they are referred to a psychiatrist, when the bubble finally bursts"

"Such patients are sent to try us. The only function they have in life is to make our lives miserable," James consoled.

"Live and let live," Rodney finished just as Elena announced dinner was ready.

James was happy with the progress of his practice and his bank manager was always delighted to see him. However he was beginning to note that his romance frontier was not advancing.

4

The available nursing currency at the hospital was decidedly too counterfeit for his liking. Janet introduced him to some of her teacher friends but to no avail. Most of them indulged in small talk which was one of his pet hates. A date with any such characters would be mentally demanding particularly if there was no substantive physical attraction. Some amends could be made for a date, but not for a lifetime. Under the circumstances he would prefer to read.

A couple of years passed and James had all the elements of a successful private practice on Bolton Street and he was quite pleased with himself. Things were going very well at the hospital as well. However he was still not seriously romantically involved yet.

One day he read an advertisement calling for volunteers for a mission trip to India for lip and cleft palate surgery by an American charity organisation. He was excited to join for a three month trip as it would provide him with new and perhaps challenging problems, he thought. He applied and was accepted. His visit would occur in the next two months and he would go to Bombay where cases would be wheeled in from the surrounds for operative management. All arrangements would be made and all reasonable expenses would paid by the organisation.

Stepping off the plane at Santacruz airport he realised that Bombay was hot and humid. The noise around was interruptive and commanded noninterpretive inattention. Everyone appeared employed physically. There was a man attempting to move a bench and another two were supervising and advising him on the mechanics of the procedure. This was obvious to James by their manual actions. When the supervisors got to what seemed like an argumentative discourse indicated by the tempo of their voices, the worker squatted and was resting.

The usual formalities obeyed he finally emerged out of the airport intending to take a taxi to JJ Hospital where he had to present himself. Outside the airport was an invasion by humanity and conquests appeared to be achieved only by the shouting voice.

He was immediately inundated with requests from the taxi drivers crowding and pushing about him each wanting to grab his attention.

"I take you very cheap sir."

"I take you there very phast sir."

"I take you …."

"I take you…."

Priorities had to be considered, choices were being offered. James was mentally very tired.

He was reminded of his arrival at Fiumichino Airport in Rome on a trip from Leeds, a few years ago. Similar turmoil prevailed. He wondered if the Indians were ancient Italians or the Italians were ancient Indians. He must read further on this one.

On this occasion he pushed himself towards one of the parked taxis and sat inside. It was now the duty of the winning driver to get the other drivers away from him which the man dutifully did with some manual and verbal intonations. The car motor started after some noisy and threatening eructations.

"Going to bhere?"

"JJ Hospital," James replied hoping he had understood the question.

"Are you doctor?"

"Yes"

"My father he pain in leg. Doctor tell him opration on back. How opration on back? Pain in leg. He see ayurvedic. He give him medicine. Pain much better."

James preferred not to intervene and nodded.

The monologue persisted as the taxi weaved its way through the noisy traffic to include motor, human, horse, bullock and donkey powered vehicles.

After much intervehicular negotiating in defiance of Newton's laws of motion, the taxi finally arrived at JJ Hospital. The hospital, inclusive of the medical school appeared to be spread over a vast compound. The taxi dropped him at the main building and the driver was paid. Two locally attired gentlemen with heavy moustaches were waiting for him at the main door. As soon as they saw him they joined their palms together and uttered, "Namaste."

James imitated them in response.

The first gentleman began, "Good morning Doctor Regan, we are bery pleased to meet you. Me, myself am Doctor Arvind Ambedkar and I am dean." Pointing to the other gentleman he continued, "This good self, himself is Doctor Mohamed Khaled and he is assistant dean. We hope you will like our hospital and your stay here. I believe you have arranged your own accommodation."

"Yes I did at a place called Breach Candy."

"You must be tired after your long journey. You can go to your accommodation. We can call you a taxi. Would you like to have dinner with my family this evening?"

"That is very kind of you Doctor Ambed. I do feel very tired. Perhaps at another time I would be delighted."

"As you wish. Shall we call a taxi?"

'That would be very nice."

James arrived at the Breach Candy apartment and found the estate agent in his labelled uniform waiting for him at the door. He introduced himself and was given the keys along with the paid invoice for his stay.

The two room apartment was furnished adequately for his needs. The initial musty smell was soon repaired by opening all the windows. James was tired. Nevertheless he took the lift down and brought some apples and bananas for dinner tonight and breakfast tomorrow.

Next morning he presented himself in the plastic surgery ward at the hospital and introduced himself to the senior registrar, Dr. Bhatt who appeared delightfully pleased to make his acquaintance and informed him that they were expecting his arrival.

"Dr Ambedkar said you will be arriving today."

"Yes, I met him yesterday," James replied.

"Would you like me to show you around hospital?"

"I'd love that."

"No problem. We go."

"Where from in Australia are you?"

"Warners Bay."

The senior registrar appeared perturbed. James had exposed a hole in his geographical knowledge of Australia which was restricted only to Sydney. Not wanting to risk opprobrium he decided not to chase the subject further.

"We have operating list this afternoon. So I will show you the operating theatres first."

"Good. Have you got much on?"

"Yes. Today is reconstruction surgery day. We have base tongue squamous cell carcinoma and neck dissection that will take all afternoon for Dr. Katekar. Then us have to do reconstruction. We have lot of oropharyngeal cancer in India because of betel nut chewing. They usually present very late as they try hope and prayer first, then homeopathy then radiotherapy and when all that no success they come to us. Most often it is too late."

"We have some of those kinds of patients too but without the betel nuts. They are just nuts in the head. Luckily not many."

This provoked a laugh from the senior registrar echoed for completion by James.

James assisted in the surgical procedure that afternoon which consisted of a mandibular visor flap to cut the mandible for access to the tumour. An elective neck dissection followed. The reconstruction was uneventful.

Soon he was able to fit in with the routine and was always an extra helping hand for the hard working residents.

During his time at the hospital he felt very sorry for the Indian resident doctors who as interns and residents were required to work a one hundred and sixty eight hour week for a measly rupee sum a year. They were on call every night and every weekend. Any time off had to be bargained for with a fellow resident. It must have been painful but under the circumstances it paid to be friends with all doctors, he thought. In addition to doing the admission history and physical examination, they also had to do the admission blood and urine analysis. There were no phlebotomists or intravenous teams. They started their own intravenous drips. The orderlies used to take patients for x-rays. Sometimes the doctors had to do that too when the orderlies were busy elsewhere. When doing Emergency roster rotation they often saw over two hundred and fifty patients a day.

Some hospital residents befriended him and showered him with advice on the sights, sounds and tastes of Bombay of which he took note. Some offered to accompany him if they could arrange their time off. James usually thanked them with a polite refusal. He could barely understand them and their incessant monologues most of the time. He noted that generally the parsi and goan residents' command of the English language was superior.

UNDOING BANDAGES: A PLASTIC NOVEL

He decided that he would get a travel agent to arrange his sightseeing trips about. The agent suggested half day leisurely periods and the first one was arranged for Victoria Terminus, a train terminal in the Fort area of Bombay on the next Sunday.

James was astonished by the Gothic style sandstone structure of the railway terminus. He did not expect such a structure here. His guide, Akbar was a middle aged man with a fascination for hair on the head, upper lip region and chin which he amply possessed and was proud to display. He had tar stained teeth in a habitat of similarly stained gums. Even his words were stained with cigarette smell. Akbar informed him that the terminus was built by the British and opened in 1887. Akbar also told him that being a railway station it was better not to get any closer, as it is possible to be carried away in the moving crowd and unless one was versed with the bearings one would be lost. James would have liked to have ventured further in but he would do it another day on his own, he thought.

Akbar read his mind, "If you want to come back here, come in the late evening. It is beautifully lighted"

"I shall do that"

Akbar suggested they visit the Gateway of India at Apollo Bunder next. On arrival Akbar pointed to James that this arched basalt structure was built to welcome King George V. James was fascinated by the structure on the waterfront overlooking the Arabian Sea which bore a Muslim style of architecture. There was entertainment provided by the roaming vendors and petty entertainers around.

Suddenly there was a tap on his shoulder, "I photo take outer. I shoot you."

Before he could understand the gravity or the ungravity of his contribution to the situation, the man produced three portrait photographs of James and handed it to him. Akbar quickly came to his rescue and urged the photographing menace to go away, in the local dialect.

"We should take a ferry to the Elephanta Caves now," Akbar offered.

"Whatever you say. You are in charge," James responded.

Ferries were available from the gateway and Akbar procured their seat tickets. The ferry was crowded both in space and with the local din. Adolescent males with heavily brylcreamed hair and a comb in their left shirt pocket dominated the boat. They reached for the comb periodically to combat any perceived piliform mutiny that may be noticed by the females in the immediate environment. The females on their part appeared not to offer any visible clues regarding their disinterest or otherwise.

It took about an hour of unspectacular spindrift water views to overcome before disembarkation on the other side and a short miniature train ride awaited them before delivery to the Caves.

The high relief cut stone sculptures were mostly damaged and shared the available accommodation with monkeys who entertained the short limbed visitors with their antics. James endured it for an hour before suggesting a return which Akbar was delighted to hear.

On the return trip, when they were approaching the Gateway to India, Akbar pointed the Taj Mahal Palace Hotel to James and mentioned that *Neil Armstrong*, the first person to walk on the moon, had stayed there. James was not sure whether he implied that the experiences would be comparable.

On disembarkation, James invited him to share a drink with him at the Taj Mahal Palace Hotel. Akbar had *ragda pattice* which is potato patties with a peas curry and chutney dish, and a *falooda* drink and James on advice from Akbar was allowed *tandoori chicken* and beer after the waiter was advised to tone down the spice in the tandoori. James enjoyed the spiced tandoori. He could live with this food and resolved to visit more Indian restaurants back home.

Akbar and James parted company after James had tipped him handsomely. James took a taxi to his apartment at Breach Candy. On the way back James reflected that he may be better on his own next time. He may need to research the places a bit. He had the time. He wished he had a paramour locally that could accompany him on these trips. How he would love that! However he calculated that the risk benefit ratio in these circumstances would be very high.

Next morning at work, Dr. Bhatt inquired, "How was trip yesterday?"
"Very good."
"Where did you go?"

"We started with Victoria Terminus, then Gateway and then Elephanta Caves"

"I never been to Elephanta Caves. Were they nice?"

"Yes."

"One day when I finish exams I will go."

"That's always the problem."

"You go to Marine Drive and Chowpatty Beach next time. Marine Drive really beautiful at night. They call it Queen's Necklace. Street lights look like string of pearls."

"Thank you for that. Maybe next Sunday."

"I would come with you. But I have study."

"I understand. I have been there before."

Next Sunday he took a taxi to Marine Drive and strolled along the promenade. He was surprised with the number of women of all shapes, sizes and skin colours with their multicoloured attires of varying types of clothing to include sarees and jeans. They travelled in waves often holding hands or with locked elbows. Ironically he remembered Samuel Coleridge's poem, *'The Rime of the Ancient Mariner'* - *'water, water everywhere and not a drop to drink'*. One such drop would suffice for him!

He returned back and went for a swim at the local public pool. Within, he attracted significant staring attention from the local males and quasi-clandestine visual attention from the passing females. Subsequently he went for an acoustically taxing walk along Warden Road. He saw several elderly British expatriates attempting to exhibit their athletic prowess by running a bit faster than the road itself! Later he had a quick vegetarian meal at a local restaurant and then off to bed.

The night was hot and relatively humid and he was forced to avail himself of the conditionally temperamental airconditioning facility.

Next morning he woke up and could not recollect his dream sufficiently. Vaguely he remembered that he was running away from *Cleopatra* or was it *Helen of Troy*? Or was it that woman in the romantic painting by *Eugène Delacroix, Liberty*? The one with the amplified breasts? He preferred Cleopatra or better still *Elizabeth Taylor*. Anyway it did not matter. The woman was threatening to kill him with a snake and he was running for his life. Perhaps it was his fascination with the snake charmers at Gateway of India that prompted this intrusion. He felt the sides of his bed and assured himself that he was safe. He would need to get out of bed soon and prepare for both his planned and mostly unplanned assignments for the day.

Finally he forced himself out of bed as the hawkers in the street below announced their wares for the day, in ever increasing loudness. He attempted to get himself ready. Already he was beginning to feel somewhat homesick. Could this be from his loneliness? He had also not slept very well with the night heat. He was glad that neck ties were not worn by the hospital resident staff routinely and he was not going to encourage them by his example now. He took a taxi to the hospital and was greeted by the registrar on arrival with an interesting case of cleft lip and palate that was due for surgery that afternoon. They discussed the possible techniques that could be employed in the situation but agreement was not in sight. Subsequently the conversation shifted and James asked, "So Dr.Bhatt what are your plans after you pass?"

"I think I will go to Amrica for more training"

"Why don't you come to Australia. I will help you"

"Thank you but no. All my friends go the Amrica and Australia is racist I heard."

"Yes that is true to an extent but it is changing."

"Okay I will think it. It also depends on I get married, which my parents want me to soon"

"How you got someone in mind?"

"No we are not allowed. The girl's father will offer dowry which I use to buy a nice flat and live. I come from a village called Wakan near Poladpur which is south of Bombay. My family will look for girl from there. I trust their choice."

James pondered Lord Tennyson's poem, *The Charge of the Light Brigade*. 'Theirs not to reason why, Theirs but to do and die'. He thought this was a form of reverse prostitution where the male gets paid. Some cultures and beliefs are difficult for outsider cultures to understand and are beyond acceptable reason and logic and sometimes even emotion, he fathomed and it was not his to reason why.

If he was Indian could he have understood? Not if he was allowed to think for himself and herein lay the deficiency he thought.

5

One day in the ward, through the periphery of his vision James saw a female figure which appeared to challenge the confines of her uniform both below and above the navel line approaching urgently towards him. Wondering what he may have done to cause this swift locomotion, he turned towards her and was delighted with the smile that she offered and reciprocated with one of his own. He had not seen her before. She has definitely upsetting his hormonal homeostasis as indicated by the dial in his groins which had moved significantly. He was besotted.

Something about her appeared to turn him on. He would analyse that factor later but now he needed verbal action.

"Hello", she began bravely, "My name is Carmen, Carmen DeCruz"

"Hi. That's a nice name. I like it. My name is James Regan. I am from Australia. I am here for a while," James rolled his tongue.

Carmen observed him rolling his tongue and decided it best to ignore it at this stage.

"I don't know much about Australia except that there are kangaroos there."

"Have you seen a real kangaroo? In Australia we find them mainly in the bush."

"Bush?"

"Yes, that's the word we use when we mean out in the country."

"Do you have bushes in the country?"

"Not necessarily, but that's the word we use."

"Hmm."

He saw his chance and quickly replied, "If you let me I will tell you all about Australia that you want to know."

She saw his move as intrusive and as goan catholic girls usually do, just walked away.

For a few seconds James pondered over what he had said that may have disturbed her. He analysed every word he had said to her with great scrutiny. Or maybe that he rolled his tongue, he thought. There was no one he could consult on the matter without inviting an adverse response for attempting to chat up local girls. There was work to do.

Later he saw her in the ward. He approached her like a frightened and confused mouse when she was alone and, "I am very sorry if I offended you earlier."

Carmen having realised the irony of her response smiled, "No, all is fine. You must tell me about Australia when you find the time."

"Sure, not a problem," he responded.

That night as he lay in bed he could not work out if he was infatuated by her or if he was in love. How does one know? After all, all his emotional indicators appeared similar as far as he could tell in this case. In his prior relationships he always had some inkling either way. Nevertheless he decided to take advantage of his propitious fortune without being committal. He would have to inveigle her into a romantic game.

He knew she would not fit in with his career motives and path just in case he was in love with her and with his family's racist tendencies, there was absolutely no chance whatsoever. Racism was a national heritage issue in friends and families he knew at home and to avoid ostracism he had cooperated with the flow although he had managed to successfully jettison it during his stay in England. He remembered incidents in school when the sons of Italian and Greek migrants were targeted. He remembered *Mariowog* as Mario was addressed, and how he had cooperated with the mob. He felt ashamed. He had read about aborigines but had no first hand experiences to relate to in this matter. He had seen some aborigines at the Royal Newcastle hospital but they usually frequented the renal and diabetic facilities. He also remembered reading that in 1835 the entire Tasmanian aboriginal population were forced into exile at the Aboriginal Establishment on Flinders Island in Bass Strait. Such incidents had made him uncomfortable within when he read about them. However with Carmen he would have to comply for his own survival.

On her way home that evening, Carmen on her part realised that she had felt different when he spoke to her. Something was not right within her since that moment. She realised that she was attracted to him. She had felt a similar sensation years before in her teenage years but the object of her desire then, a certain Joseph Carvalho, had been usurped by the local Catholic clergy army which uses a 'guilt you' technique to recruit young needy innocents with assurance of a free bed, meals and higher catholic education in catholic institutions in exchange for a lifetime of devotion and celibacy. Joseph had departed without even letting her know. She felt the sensation this time was much stronger and looked forward to engaging with James fruitfully soon, hopefully tomorrow.

Next day James mustered enough courage to ask Carmen for a movie and dinner date. He had home worked the attitude of the catholic families to romance and particularly with white foreigners and was prepared for a refusal. However she appeared delighted and after the initial expected polite hesitancy finally accepted his offer to meet him at the Kit Kat Restaurant and later to Metro Cinema at Dhobi Talao to watch the movie, *"Send me no flowers"* with *Rock Hudson* and *Doris Day*.

Things were beginning to happen for him. He arrived early and waited outside the restaurant and was promptly molested by the on duty beggars. He had not learned that awarding a coin to one was a recipe to invite an avalanche with kaleidoscopic deformities.

Carmen arrived soon after dressed in a magnificent cerulean salwar kameez which is the traditional dress of Punjabi women and he was rescued promptly with her cries of *"hatto"* which he learnt later meant "move away".

They went into the restaurant and were escorted to a booth with a single table and seats, by a waiter and supplied with the drink and food menu. The lighting had been dimmed to create a romantic atmosphere. Several oil paintings of local flora adorned the walls. James' eyes honed in on the marigolds, "I love marigolds."

"Me too," Carmen reciprocated.

"Do you know why they are called marigolds?"

"No. Why?"

"The word comes from Mary's gold after the virgin."

"Really."

"In Spain they were placed on the altar of Mary."

"Interesting."

"That's a lotus flower," James pointed to another painting.

Carmen directed her sight towards the direction of his pointing finger, "Yes. That's a very special flower for our spiritual India. Because the lotus flower rises from the mud without stains, they are often considered as a symbol of purity. Some think that that the lotus flower is a symbol representing the transcending of man's spirit over worldly matter since it blooms from the underworld into the light. It is a symbol of the divine in Hinduism, Buddhism Jainism and Sikhism."

"We get lotuses also in Queensland in Australia where the climate is also conducive for their growth."

"Is Queensland to the north or south of Sydney?"

"North. Anyway you better make your choices before the waiter comes back."

"I am no good with alcohol choices. I will have

whatever you are having," Carmen said.

"And I'm no good with the food choices here. I will have whatever you are having," he said.

"You will be sorry."

"I have been sorry before," he echoed as he was reminded of his encounter at a Indian restaurant in Sheffield, England when he braved the chilli code and was punished without mercy at both ends on separate days. Hopefully it would be worth it on this occasion.

"Would you be comfortable with a kingfisher beer? I shall leave the food choices to you."

"Yeah I will have a beer. Also tell me, where in Australia do you come from?" she inquired.

"I come from a place called Warners Bay. It is north of Sydney on the east coast of Australia."

"I have some distant maternal relations in Perth. We never hear from them," she added.

After a while she asked, "What religion are you?"

"I am roman catholic but I am an atheist."

"How can that be? Isn't being an atheist and a catholic mutually exclusive?" she retorted.

"Being catholic is a lineage and a culture. The religion is distinct."

She saw his point of view. Considering her own situation she realised that she had some thinking to do on the subject.

"We need to talk about this another time. I want to know more. Let us resolve to just enjoy today." She realised that she was also mentally attracted to him. She wanted to be a part of his life. She wanted a part of him. However that may not be possible in her present status. But one never knows.

"Well said" he replied.

The movie theatre was a welcome relief from the extreme heat outside. As they settled on their seats he reached out and held her hand. However she did not object as he had expected. Of course kissing in an Indian theatre was socially prohibited and even in the darkness there are always prying eyes which can instigate a mob to attempt to disrupt one's anatomy and particularly that of a of a foreigner dating a local girl. He remembered *Cliff Richard's "Andole Y 'Arriva"* and did not wish for that fate.

As she was attempting to follow the movie she was interrupted by her fast heart beats which she tried to ignore consciously but to no avail. She felt herself hopelessly not in control.

After the movie he suggested that they get some ice cream at the Harvic restaurant next to Kit Kat restaurant across the road.

"What a good idea. You are exceptionally brilliant today," she humoured.

"It runs in the family," he winked trying to keep the humour going.

Attempting to part the traffic with a raised hand in the like of the fabled Moses and the Red Sea episode is like inviting the red sea within oneself to erupt with a few broken bones thrown in for good measure and completion, he thought. Nevertheless, they crossed the road which was mostly a death defying experience for him.

She ordered *mango lassi* and he ordered vanilla ice cream.

They discussed the movie. Both of them liked it.

"That Kingfisher beer we had earlier. I liked it. We have some interesting beer in Australia too."

"I don't know much about beer. For us it is quite recent after all the prohibition years."

"Did you know that beer has been drunk for eight thousand years. In fact the survival of some communities in years gone by can be traced to the fact that they drank beer rather than water, which was contaminated with pathogens. Brewing of beer includes a boiling stage that destroys harmful organisms."

"We could have done with some beer in our cholera days. I am sure some of our patients would love that but there would be always be some who would rather choose to die rather than consume alcohol," Carmen added.

"For all beers, we can consider their quality, their color, whether they are hazy or not, their foam, and their flavour. The many attributes of beer depend on the palette of malted grains and hops that are used to make them, as well as the yeast and water used."

"Like cooking a good old curry it seems."

"Indeed. Beer or ale, as it would have been in those days, was the drink for all times of day, including breakfast, lunch, and dinner. Much of the history of brewing started in the British Isles. Beer is made from four main raw materials: grain, hops, yeast, and water. The main grain that is used worldwide is barley. There are two types of hops - bittering hops which have very high levels of resins and aroma hops which have great aromas. Water of course can be classified in terms of their hardness, as soft and hard. There are two types of brewing yeast. Ale yeast and lager yeast."

"That's' interesting," Carmen lied.

"Lambic beers are a famous Belgian-style product which is sour. These types of beers are made with different types of microorganisms. These beers are not available everywhere. Some people add fruit to beer. Cherries, raspberries peaches, apples and blackcurrant. Shandy is half ale and half lemonade. Coriander and chilli sometimes find their way in too. I read that Kingfisher like other lagers is made from a combination of barley, rice, and flaked corn."

"Really?"

All this was not information Carmen particularly wanted to know. However she had to provide the 'Wow, That's interesting' look. She did not wish to sound impolite. She could not afford it. She wanted this relationship to sail. Hoping to terminate the subject she offered, "I am interested in your religion views James."

"I am an atheist. So I have no views on the subject," he responded

"You know what I mean," she laughed

"But that's for another date," he chided

"Okay" she retorted happy that another date was in the offing.

He realised his moves were working well and he may get far with her. However he did not wish to push too quickly.

"Can I see you home?"

"No, that will not be needed. I can get an A4 bus

from right here to drop me in front of where I live in Byculla on Clare Road near Gloria Church."

"I think I know where that is." He was reminded of the gothic structure which was initially built by the Portuguese that he had seen in his prior excursions of the area.

"My family attends that church every Sunday."

"Is your family very devout?" He needed to know.

"Yes within the bounds of neighbourly gossip," she laughed.

"I suppose that's a universal catholic trait."

James did not wish to push this further. He knew that some people liked to talk about their families till the listener developed tinnitus from repetition of the same chorus of information and others do not like to talk about their families for reasons that may allow public interpretation. Either way it is always safe to refrain from inquisitivity.

"Its getting late. I better go home. I have to iron my uniform."

"What time do you start tomorrow?" James queried.

"Seven."

"I better let you go then. I will see you at work tomorrow and don't be late."

"Not a chance," she retorted.

They left the restaurant with James following behind. The vulpine beggars spotted him but soon remembered their earlier unproductive effort and allowed him to depart in a passing taxi. Carmen having assured herself that her efforts would not be required to rescue him from his proness to beggars tendency went towards her own bus stop.

On his way back in the taxi James pondered on his success and complimented himself on a fruitful evening with further prospects awaiting. Carmen on her part was especially buoyant. Her father Porfiro, who had been a train driver had died about five years ago of a heart attack would be very proud of her if she was successful in procuring a marriage without a dowry and her mother who had not recovered from his memory would definitely be happy. Her brother Cecil, having obtained a science degree was a pharmaceutical representative with Merck Sharp and Dohme and usually concurred with her in all matters, whether safe or unsound. He would definitely be happy in this case, at least for the mere financial reason.

6

The next day was Saturday and at the hospital she avoided him and his gaze to disarouse co-worker suspicion. James was puzzled and thought she had decided against his advances. Did I do or say something wrong? He set about the task of analysing the conversation and his deeds yesterday. He could not fault himself, no matter how hard he tried. He was at a loss to understand. However he could not let this opportunity go unassailed. In fact he felt he was doing quite well here, he thought. He resolved to do whatever was required. He watched her closely and when she was alone approached her.

"Hello Carmen, how are you today?"

"Very good and you?"

"Top of the world. Are you trying to avoid me?" he asked.

"Not at all. Just avoiding suspicion and gossip."

"Can we meet again?"

"That depends on you," she replied.

"Here's my telephone. Ring me after six tonight," and he handed her a piece of paper.

"Will do," Carmen replied grabbing the paper and quickly putting it in her uniform pocket and walking away.

That evening, precisely at six, Carmen rang him.

"Hello James, how are you?"

"Wrapped in thoughts about you. Can you come

over? We can go out."

"Sure. Give me your address."

"Have you got a piece of paper?"

Carmen was already equipped, "Fire on."

"Flat five, Forty six Warden Road, Breach Candy. I am on the third floor. Take the lift I will be waiting for you."

She arrived by taxi to Warden Road and took the lift up to his apartment and rang the bell.

He opened the door and welcomed her in with a tight kiss.

Carmen was thrilled. She had never been kissed before and she had a lot to learn from this maestro.

His apartment had a lounge room with a sofa set and some vedic mythology books on the floor, two bedrooms, kitchen and toilet and was minimally furnished.

He was dressed and waiting and she suggested to him that they go to Gaylords at Churchgate. He agreed.

They went down and hailed a taxi to Churchgate.

James was amazed by the automotorbatics of the local drivers. However, such tactics were not for him. The taxi dropped them at Gayords and James settled the adulterated meterage amount with the driver who offered to wait for him if required. James thanked him and let him go.

Gaylord was located on the main street at Churchgate with several other eating places around.

At Gaylords, they were escorted to a table and

Carmen ordered coconut water and he asked for a coca cola. On instructions from her, they chose the tandoori option meals with Carmen threateningly informing the waiter to keep it very low in pungency.

After the meal James complimented her choices and asked for the names of the dishes.

"Can I pay?" she inquired.

"Not on your life." he replied.

She was not keen to instigate a nugatory scene and walked towards the door whilst James settled the account.

Later, they walked to the Parsi Diary Farm and partook of some ice cream.

They strolled along Marine drive enjoying the mild sea breeze and were very soon accompanied by the wandering mendicants. Carmen took over and made them disperse pell-mell.

They decided to sit on the parapet backing Back Bay and the Arabian Sea. He held her hand.

"Let us continue the conversation from last time James."

"What was that about, remind me."

"Tell me about your religious beliefs."

"I have no religious beliefs. End of story," he responded

"How did you come to that conclusion?"

"Some time ago, I really and firmly believed in all that Christian mysticism. Suddenly I realised that I believed things that I had not checked upon myself. A sort of *René Descartes* moment! The more I thought about it, the more it did not make sense. Angels coming from heaven, virgins giving birth, people being raised from the dead, three gods in one, an infallible pope, all just pure crap. These early church fathers, knowing the insane gullibility of the age, set their wits to work in the imagination of improbable possibilities and odd accidents. We are must better informed now. If Jesus had really performed miracles do you think the Jews would let go of him from their religion?"

Carmen was lost in thought. What James said made so much sense. She needed to think about it for her own sake. One can't go through a lifetime believing ancient traditions.

James persisted, "By all history records, Pontius Pilate was a very cruel man. The Christian church fathers do not allow him so in their story. In my opinion if the holocaust had not occurred in living memory, these church fathers would probably have made up a story that Hitler was a nice man and the holocaust did not happen. The Romans buried crucified criminals in mass graves. This is a fact in the Roman history records. But of course to resurrect Jesus, you need a private tomb and so the story was made to accommodate this. The Christians merely took a dead Jew and made a god of him. Does this make sense to you?"

"But that is the power of God"

"Yes, he is god because he has the power and because he has the power he is god. It is just a circular argument. Like you would say it is red because its an apple and it's an apple because its red." He was trying to make it comprehensible to Carmen. He continued, "If you read carefully Emperor Constantine called the Nicean Council in Nicaea, to actually vote for Jesus as God. Imagine being voted as God. We do that with Presidents and Prime Ministers these days but we don't worship them." This was beyond Carmen. She did not know that Jesus' case was settled by voting, a little known fact! And well hidden by the Byculla clergy! Or did they themselves actually know it? They did not care. It provided them with a living.

"Do you think evolution is true? Of course it is. We now have comparative biological, fossil and DNA evidence and who knows in future we may get some more types of proof.

"I have no problem with evolution," Carmen said.

"If we are descended from apes then where does Adam and Eve fit in?"

"Adam and Eve is only a metaphoric story to explain sin," Carmen repeated as was ingrained in her by the local frocked clerics.

"Then sin came into the world from a metaphoric story. And Jesus died for a metaphoric story? No Carmen, sin is our evolved tendency to be greedy and selfish to survive in this competitive world. And if god made us like that, then he is responsible for sin."

The topic was now beginning to hurt Carmen's conscious mind.

"Yes, what you say is possibly true. But I need to think more about it."

"Remember, religion tells you what to think, you need to know how to think. And finally isn't which religion you accept and which you reject really accidents of your own birth?"

Carmen was lost in thought. She realised that this was happening on her own provocation of James but what James said made sense. After all, when did she ever subject her religion to any real thinking of her own? It was all based on her emotions and views provided by others. Particularly those individuals whose livelihood depended on it.

He continued further, "After much reading on the subject. I have realised that the church has misled us with fairy tales to include subjects like the trinity, original sin, immaculate conception, papal infallibility and the like. It was okay in ancient times when people were gullible and science did not exist and evidence was not required. The main culprit here was Paul, not the apostle but the guy who was on his way to persecute the Christians and fell off his horse as he was perhaps dozing and had a hallucination. If you look at religions you will note that the Jewish god is punitive and demands a master slave relationship with his selected followers. The Catholic god used to be punitive but has matured and mellowed over the years. This god is now sympathetic within bounds. The Muslim god demands a passive aggressive response from followers."

It appeared that Carmen was cracking, "In India being in the spiritual tradition that is imposed on us all, the contradicting literature is hidden away just like in olden times the church tried to burn all the works of Aristotle and nearly succeeded, but for the Muslims."

"It is interesting how the various civilisations adopted different cultural systems, the Chinese picked bureaucracy, the Indians chose spirituality generating Hinduism and Buddhism and the Greco-Romans found a theoretical route. Ultimately culture, is the sense of basic beliefs, values, and assumptions and is a vital part of the human experience," James added.

"I suppose we humans have to rely on culture because we do not have many basic instincts," Carmen added.

"That is an interesting observation Carmen. All the great thinkers like *Confucius, Lao Tzu, Zoroaster* and *Buddha* were already present much before Christ. The Bible is essentially copied from Plato's thoughts if you look at it closely," James continued.

"Yes, I agree. Please let us close on that for now," Carmen had had enough of religion for the moment. She resolved to think more about it in her own time.

"You started it Carmen. I have done very significant reading on the Christian religion before rejecting it as absolute total myth."

"In India we use our spirituality mostly to implore the Almighty to give us enough strength to endure the misfortunes of others," Carmen humoured and this provoked a laugh from James.

He was also beginning to appreciate her sense of humour. He could do with some during his stay here.

"What shall we talk about now?" James inquired.

"Tell me James. I am really amazed with your knowledge. You know so much. How come?"

"My father is an ear nose throat surgeon. From an early age I learnt that there was no place for small talk in my entire family. He set about the task of educating us by inciting the curiosity of our young minds so our conversations would be more fruitful.

He knew that young minds are like sponges for knowledge. Our conversations were only informative. Idle gossip was strictly forbidden by both my parents. Even now I can't stand any such gossip. Also I read as much as I can. So there you are. You are hereby warned."

"How wise of your parents."

"I remember the day my father taught me how to appreciate art."

"I always thought that art was inherent."

"Techniques may be but appreciation can be learnt. When you look at a work it is important to first note the point of view, which is where the viewer stands in relationship to the scene depicted."

"You mean from above, below, or straight on. Right?"

"Right. Next the focal point which is the main focus of a work of art, the place where your eye will almost automatically land on your first viewing. Next note the colour theme whether primary, secondary or tertiary and their combinations whether analogous or complementary."

"I learnt colours in primary school. I know what you mean."

"Next note how the artist has depicted his lines whether they are descriptive and defining the object's outline, whether they are curved or mathematical. Next the shapes which may again be curved or mathematical. Generally mathematical shapes are stable but curved are livelier. Next how does the artist show space?"

"He uses perspective right?"

"One way. Other ways are shading and overlapping."

"Tell me about chiaroscuro. I have heard that word often."

"The use of black pigment to create these effects is chiaroscuro. Caravaggio is a master of this. Finally texture is also created by using light. Hard objects reflect light and soft objects absorb light."

"Rocks will reflect light and feathers will absorb," Carmen understood.

"Spot on Carmen."

"Thank you. I'm getting better at this."

"Composition is the combination of colour, line, shape that provide a work of art a sense of balance."

"Interesting," Carmen was learning and was impressed by James' explanations.

"Of course paintings can be made in various media like water colours, oils, gouache etcetera. And paintings may be landscapes or portraits which may again be realistic, idealised, distorted or abstracted."

"That's very nice. Thank you James."

"Plenty more from where that came."

"Don't I know?" she reached out and held his hand tight. Wouldn't it be nice to spend one's whole life with this man? He has so much to offer. And he is so willing to part with his knowledge.

"You should spend some time in an art gallery and practice more."

"Unfortunately we do not have any paintings from any great artists here."

"Although great artists like Leonardo, Caravaggio, Vermeer teach us many things, all artists are important in their own way, if you learn to appreciate art. Indian art has a long history, I am sure."

"Sorry I don't know much about Indian art but I will make it my business to do so from now on.

Thank you for guiding me into that."

"That's exactly my business Carmen. To incite curiosity. In fact the more you know a subject the more enjoyable it becomes, That's what I found. Knowledge should be shared unselfishly. Don't you think?"

"Of course. Tell me something about European artists," Carmen said.

"What do you know already?"

"Not much."

"Art in Europe is divided into periods, initiating with Romanesque followed by Gothic and then Medieval. Remember these are not fixed periods with lots of overlapping. Medieval art is iconic and is abstracted with generic faces. The subjects are religious and supernatural. Next we have Early Renaissance where the figure is more individual and human. However they are not realistic and the proportions are inconsistent. Dutch renaissance brings in oils and pictures of everyday life. High Renaissance introduces geometric compositions and perspective. The human figure is better. Baroque painting has intense drama and strong diagonals. The subjects are mainly royalty. *El Greco* produces Mannerism with distorted proportions, size and even perspective. Southern Baroque celebrates the Church and French Baroque celebrates Louis XIV. Dutch Baroque has portraits, still life and Old Testament stories. Rococo has curves and cupids in the lives of aristocrats." James stopped and wanted time to refresh his memory.

"What's the matter?" Carmen asked.

"No, just wondering if I have missed anything."

"Have you?"

"No. Next comes Neoclassicism with closed compositions and stoic contents followed by Romanticism which is really baroque with high drama and exotic worlds.

Next we have Realism with *Manet* which is real world. Impressionism followed with *Monet* and the Postimpressionism with *van Gogh* followed by expressionism which aims for psychological empathy. And can you guess who comes next?"

"No."

"Cubism."

"*Picasso*?" Carmen attempted to guess.

"Yes."

"I love Picasso."

"My father likes Picasso too. He says he can watch it all day and not understand a thing."

"I agree with your father."

"Basically cubism portrays a three dimensional form on a two dimensional surface with multiple points of view," James continued.

"Never thought of it that way."

"Next follows Abstract art with *Pollock* and Surrealism with *Salvador Dali* and Postmodernism and pop art with *Andy Warhol*. The end."

"That was very nice and most interesting"

"The ideas of the ancient Greek and Romans were important for the understanding of art during the Renaissance. The pursuit of beauty was considered by the ancients as the highest goal of art. This idea was inherited by the Renaissance, especially in Italy. The goal of art changed throughout the centuries for most artists, turning from beauty toward something that could express the experiences of real life. Ancient thinkers, such as *Socrates, Plato, Aristotle* and *Cicero*, singled out specific qualities for praise which influenced artists and writers in later centuries. Among them are composition harmony and proportion.

Art like music is individual and can never be an entirely rational task, because there are no universal objective rules for judging or for producing quality or beauty in art.

Also don't forget that artists are conditioned mostly by circumstances beyond their actual control. During the earlier times, most art of the highest level was made on commission. From the beginning of the sixteenth century the number of works of art not made on commission and just for the open market began to grow, changing the dynamics of how artists could make money for their work. Where neither the Court nor the Church were important sources of patronage, as was the case in Amsterdam in the seventeenth century, painters such as *Rembrandt* relied on the patronage of civil institutions such as militia companies and on private collectors."

"It's amazing that art is controlled by outside forces," Carmen expressed surprise. She was not aware of this aspect of art creation before.

"Louis XIV usually dictated what was good and bad taste, through the control of academies where painting and sculpture were taught."

"I learnt a lot today. I wish I had a notebook." Carmen laughed.

"You can get all that from a decent book on the History of Art."

"I will look for one."

"Ask for *Gombrich*. That's a good one."

"Give me the name later."

"Okay."

"It is getting a bit chilly. Should we go home?" she asked

"If you think so. Would you like to come over to my place?" he asked

She thought for a moment before replying, "Okay"

They got up and went in search of a taxi.

Things are going good, Carmen thought. He is so well informed in such diverse topics and is so clever. He seems to remember many things almost in detail. I have never met anyone like him to date. I hope he likes me.

7

The sun had had enough of humanity on this segment of its sojourn for the day and was deciding an unplanned boondoggle on the horizon. The clouds watched for a while and then decided to move on in the opposite direction. The street lights were already on, and the day time hawking vocalists attempting to hog the limelight during the day had retired for the night.

Up at the apartment, "I have a bottle of Johnny Walker whiskey. Would you like to try some?" James asked.

"I have never tasted it before. Yes I will try some," Carmen replied.

James fetched his bottle of Johnny Walker Blue and poured some in two drinking glasses.

"Would you like ice or soda in your drink?" James asked.

"Whatever you are having."

"I like mine neat. Nothing added.'"

"Okay. I will follow you."

He handed her a glass. "Cheers" they clinked their glasses.

Carmen sipped, "This is my first time with whiskey. I like it."

"Good. Johnny Walker is a scotch whiskey made from malted barley, while bourbon whiskey is made from corn. Bourbon comes from North America. Whiskeys are aged in wooden casks and have a minimum of forty percent alcohol. If you like it there's always more," James responded.

"Goans usually drink feni which is the local drink. It is made from coconut. Feni can also be made from cashew."

"Is it nice?"

"Very potent."

"I must try it then."

When she had finished, James asked, "Shall I pour you some more?"

"No please don't. I already feel very tipsy. I am not a great drinker, like most goans."

"You can stay here tonight if you wish," James offered, definitely expecting a negative reply.

Carmen decided that this was a much safer option than going home in a taxi. Her mother would smell the alcohol and then be offering her dispiriting comments all evening and for several months later. Her choice was thus limited.

"I have to ring home and tell them I am staying at a friend's place."

"You know where the phone is."

Carmen had never spent a night with a man alone. The consequences of such were never considered in her family as the probability of such an occurrence were deemed non-existent until after marriage. She wondered what would happen. She had no experience to go by. She decided that she would take it as it comes, as under the current circumstances she had no other choice. It was too late to alter her decision. Besides, James is a gentleman. He will not hurt me.

The initially desultory conversation drifted towards goan culture and she informed him that her family came from Goa.

"Goa is India's smallest state. It is located on the west coast, south of here. Early Goa belonged to the Mauryan empire of Emperor Ashoka. The Hindu dynasties controlled Goa for the next seven hundred years. Next came the Muslim invasion of Goa by the Bahamini Kingdom. The discovery of a new sea route to India around the Cape of Good Hope by Vasco da Gama provided the Portuguese impetus. Under the command of their Alfonso de Albuquerque Goa was colonised. The Portuguese left a significant influence on the architecture, food and education in Goa. The first missionaries to arrive were the Dominican Friars who came as chaplains of the Fleet on Albuquerque's ships. The next group was the Franciscans, The most successful group to arrive soon after were the Jesuits."

"It is amazing that these groups did not fight with each other for pride of place. Or maybe they did?"

"We will never know. The Pope would have dictated the exact terms with his usual associated threats of noncompliance."

"And the Pope is infallible. Right?"

"Yes. Christian converts were favoured in the appointments of goans to public office and some positions were even reserved for these new converts. The Portuguese also implemented the compulsory learning of the Portuguese language. Later under Dr. Antonio de Salazar's dictatorship in Portugal many goan freedoms were rescinded. Many goans, discouraged by this sudden and unexpected reversal, emigrated to Bombay. The Portuguese colonised Goa for four hundred and fifty years. The British took nearly one hundred years to conquer India and then ruled for another one hundred years. My family emigrated to Bombay in search of employment like the other goans here today. Some of my father's family left for Tanzania in Africa. We hardly hear from or about them. Some goans sought employment in merchant shipping in the culinary sections as goans are very good cooks."

James listened intently. At the mention of British rule he remembered how Ireland was oppressed by the British for more than seven hundred years. He remembered reading something in James Joyce's *Dubliners*.

"Ireland has a similar history of exploitation by the British," he said.

"I know, but I don't know the details," Carmen was aware.

That was enough to get James going.

"The Normans first came to Ireland in the seventh century. In the twelfth century, King Henry II invaded Ireland to establish English rule in Ireland. The Irish lived as part of the English, and then British Empire for over seven hundred years.

As the English nation grew in power and influence it suppressed Ireland's culture and also forced the population to speak the English language. Suppression of catholic revolts by the English and forcible incorporation of Ireland took place in in the early nineteenth century. The Irish state came into being in the early twentieth century as the 32 county Irish Republic. The territory that became Northern

Ireland had a Protestant majority who wanted to maintain ties to Britain. To counter the growing disorder surrounding civil rights protests and an increase in sectarian violence during the traditional Protestant marching season, the British Government ordered the deployment of troops to Northern Ireland in August 1969.

The British Isles now contain two sovereign states: Ireland and the United Kingdom of Great Britain and Northern Ireland.The Irish have considerable Norman and Viking ancestry in their blood – just like the British."

"Yet in India I think we need to be grateful to the British at least for taking away *sati* where widows were forced to jump in the burning pyres of their husbands."

"That would be unimaginably terrible," James expressed his horror.

"We have to be grateful to the British for that. They also invested in our railway infrastructure and promulgated allopathic medical and technological knowledge in our country. They established the seeds for democratic institutions and judicial systems in India. But as the great English bard *William Shakespeare* says *'The evil that men do lives after them. The good is oft interred with their bones.'* Most ungrateful people are conditioned that way. In India this mob mentality is referred to as nationalism and patriotism and anger against the British is thus cultivated," Carmen continued.

"*Aristotle* articulating his Principle of Moderation

states that anyone can become angry. That's easy. But to be angry at the right person and to the right degree and at the right time and for the right purpose and the right way that's not within everybody's power and that's not easy and that is really the appropriate fashion that when our passions are cultivated in the right context, they bring us happiness. Having said that I must admit I am also very deficient here," James admitted.

"The anger is labelled as patriotism. Here in India with the retreat of the British Empire and the displacement of the local landholding aristocracies we have a new kind of professional middle class," Carmen continued.

The discussion was getting more thought provoking and would contribute to sleep deprivation, if continued. On this note James suggested that it was getting late and that they should go to bed.

"The bedroom is the last room on the left. You go first," James said.

"I need to go to the toilet first."

"You know where that is."

Carmen felt a bit uncomfortable undressing in his bedroom. However she thought that one as to be pragmatic and not let emotions overrule the situation.

Carmen felt good to be in bed with him. She was confused with her body's reaction and particularly in the groin regions. She had never felt like this before. He reached out and felt her breasts. This caused her even more confusion. He came closer and kissed her hard on her lips. Carmen responded. He kissed her nipples. Carmen was beginning to lose control of her emotions. Much against her catholic grain her hands almost by reflex moved to his groins. He attempted to pull down her underwear and she lent him a helping hand with the mechanics of the garment, whenever he paused. She liked what was happening. Before long he was inside her. It was quite painful for her but very pleasant she noted. She was enjoying the feeling as he moved in and out. Suddenly he stopped and dropped out. She felt the abruptness of his action as he fell on to her side. She was lost for words as she felt she had contributed to this reaction from him. She felt she had done something wrong.

"Was that good for you?" he murmured.

"Yes very nice," she replied

Soon he fell asleep and was snoring

Carmen retraced her memory of the incident and had discombobulated thoughts. She argued it was a very pleasant feeling. So also felt guilty at losing her catholic virginity. But this had to happen sooner or later, she consoled herself. She loved him and hopefully he loved her too. But what the heck? She loved it and would do it again. With these thoughts she soon fell asleep.

She woke up early as usual and attended to her toilet needs. She still felt somewhat sore in her genitals. It was her off day at the hospital and she was in no hurry. She got back into bed with James who had not woken up yet. She thought about last night.

Was this act a rudderless drift for her into

ignominy? Such inchoate reflections did not seek any reification in her mind. She resolved that it was now in the past and nothing she could do now could rectify it. She had a winning card and under the circumstances, she can't call it quits. She will go ahead and deal with her badgering Christian mind just like James had done with his. After all he seemed to be informed.

Okay James, here I come with you to the fires of hell where there will be gnashing of teeth! What intrigued her most now was how her disembodied soul might feel the fires of hell! She was learning how to think. She was coming out of her catholic bandages and her entire body was now beginning to breathe.

James woke up some time later with a smile on his face as he saw her, "Good morning."

"Good morning to you too."

"Did you sleep okay with my snoring?"

"Did you snore? I did not hear you. Maybe I fell asleep too."

"Give me a tick and we go down for breakfast but you can make yourself a coffee in the meantime if you like." James got out from the bed.

"I'm okay. I can wait," Carmen replied.

When he had finished they walked down the road to a breakfast place. She preferred a *dosa and chutney* and he asked for fried eggs and toast and coffee.

"No religion talk today," she humoured.

"I think I have bored you enough on that subject," he replied

"No, no its not boring at all. Your discourses have made me think more than I have ever, if ever, thought about what I believe. Here in Bombay all the contradictory literature is not available to us. Our clergy keep it well away from us. Goa, from where my family comes, has a lot of crucifixes of different sizes all over the place as reminders of impending doom. It is not possible to walk any significant distance in Goa, entertaining a pleasant thought without encountering a crucifix to catapult one back to the "guilt plane" and particularly if "guilt" has been harnessed into our young minds from early childhood. Guilt entrenchment is the prime job of our clergy, by employing a calculated distortion of facts with fiction. Inquiry by a person into the occurrence of any natural phenomenon which the priest guys cannot explain is explained as an "act of God" with the result that any further inquiry is thus discouraged and if persisted in, results in a forced obliteration of the person's presence. In a sense it is considered a blasphemous desire to want to know more. If a person persists further, particularly in matters of faith than these priest guys would immediately impart instructions to pray to God to protect one from all such thoughts. Other accompanying companions would be told to be wary of such an undesirable corrupt mind. Our parents were also prey to this mass farce. My parents did not and my mother still does not understand. I must admit that I was in the same boat till you got me thinking. So I have decided that I am coming to hell with you."

James continued, "Young children are in no position to tell fact from fiction and are therefore obliged to take whatever they are told at face value. Because there is almost no limit to what little children will believe, the onus falls upon parents to ensure that children are given the tools to tell fact from fiction, proof from propaganda, and honest inquiry from wishful thinking."

The conversations were interpreted by Carmen as an ostensible indication from James regarding how they will bring up their offspring and she was in total agreement with his views.

James was not in love with her, perhaps just infatuated. By now he worked out that Carmen was an interlocutory in his life. His family would never forgive him and she would not be acceptable in his circle back in Australia. She would be an impediment to his career. After all, his career was all he had worked for all his life to date. He could not allow her to enter into his life on a more permanent basis.

He was reminded of *Billy Joel*'s *Virginia* in *"Only the good die young"* and he certainly could do with a catholic fling at this stage in this town.

She appeared available during his stay in Bombay to satisfy his sexual arousals. So why should he care as long as she agrees?

Although their first sexual encounter was brief, as first encounters usually are, he worked out that he may have been too excited at the opportunity and she may have been attempting to admonish her catholic acquired guilt. Next time he resolved that it would be slow and better.

Their sexual encounters were now more frequent and James was always the perfect gentleman. No attempt at contraception was ever mentioned by either.

James was enamoured by her skin unctuosity and colour and enjoyed the skin to skin rapport. She also looked very much forward to his advances.

Further such encounters were more protracted and more pleasant and contraception was neglected and completely ignored. Under the circumstances Carmen justified to herself that their exploits necessitated that all caution be thrown to the wind. How the mind can provide justification in any circumstance!

Sometimes Carmen did ponder what would happen if she fell pregnant. At such times she consoled herself. No point worrying about things that may never happen. She would worry about that when it actually happened. At times she thought that it would be good to have James' baby. She was enjoying the right now, right now and looked forward to sex every time they met. Before long sex was the most favoured item on the agenda. James could not believe how his fortunes had changed.

8

The inevitable of course happened and she missed her next menstrual period. It dawned on her what this may mean. There was nothing arcane. But this is meant to happen to others not me, she thought. How could I have been so stupid? No she was not stupid. Attempting to get contraceptives would have been an impossible mission for her. And she could not afford to lose James.

The real worry had now begun. What now? She thought for a while. Really there is nothing to worry about. She had James she could depend upon. He would never let her down. Particularly when it is his own baby. I wonder what the baby would look like. I just hope he or maybe she has James' skin colour and eye colour. The child would look great. Everyone would envy her. Particularly Neera and Ramona who could be relied upon to be her life long enemies. When James' term at the hospital finishes she would suggest that she go with him to Australia and perhaps have the delivery there. The hospitals there would be far superior and clean. She was sure James' parents would assist her with the delivery. How happy would they be with their first grandchild? What would her own mother, Felicity think when she finds out? She will be proud that her daughter would marry a white doctor. After all, how many can achieve that in Byculla? How I wish dad was alive. He would be so so happy. She was sure her brother Cecil would also be delighted when he is told. Such thoughts occupied her mentation incessantly. She was feeling very buoyant.

She rang for an appointment at Breach Candy Hospital and was able to secure one that afternoon. Luckily she was rostered off duty for that day. She did not seek help at her own hospital for fear of gossip at the workplace. And besides, Breach Candy Hospital was closer to James' apartment that she hoped to move into soon.

On arrival there she noted that Breach Candy Hospital appeared relatively newly built. A solitary crow sitting on the steps greeted her with requests for spare food. On noting that its attempts were proving futile it flew away.

The hospital floors were clean although not deprived of the usual hospital odour to which she was already acclimated. The nurses in their recently laundered uniforms appeared keen to exhibit the magnitude of the contained contents with a Galilean vertical pendular motion as they walked along in an impended hurry although eventually, most of the dimensions of the proposed exhibits would statistically lie towards the left end of the *Bell curve*. Nevertheless it is possible that *Galileo* would have considered his time better spent studying motion in these surrounds than in a church pew.

Carmen found the hospital directions difficult to interpret but with repeated requisitions for help along the way which were mostly misleading as expected, the out patients department was finally sighted. The requisite personal information was obtained by the staff at the outpatient reception desk and after having been asked to be poorer by parting with a few hundred rupees, she was asked to find a seat, most of which appeared to be occupied by relations and friends of the patients, with some patients even squatting on the floor with vomit bowls in hand. After a wait of at least two hours she was seen by a white coat clad doctor who identified himself as Dr. Shinde. Perhaps for the benefit of his deaf clients he also had his identity verified on his coat pocket.

After the required questioning and tampering with pelvic contents, she was requested to provide an urine sample. She tested positive to a pregnancy test.

"I am to inform you currently that you are with baby," he smiled at her as if he was already aware of her prior activity required for this result.

"Are you sure?"

"I am more than hundred percent sure of that. I myself will personally refer you to the antenatal clinic at this hospital. It is on the next floor up. You can take the lift at the end of this corridor on the left side."

He toyed with the phone at his desk and an appointment was secured for her in the next week.

Now what? The morning's buoyancy was waning. Should she not have known better to have avoided this? How is she to tell James? How will he respond? Hopefully he will take charge. He seems like the kind of person to do so anyhow.

As she was departing, suddenly she heard her name called from behind. Instinctively she looked back and recognised a nursing friend from past years. Sheena was a nurse from Kerala in the south of India who had trained with Carmen and had initially worked at JJ Hospital. She had long black hair that reeked of coconut oil.

"What brings you to Breach Candy Hospital?"

"I have had some bleeding from below," Carmen had an impromptu reply.

"Front or back?" such details had to be known for a corridor diagnosis.

"Front."

"It could be fibroids. My mother had to have a hysterectomy for that."

"The doctor does not know yet. We have to have a few tests yet."

"How is everybody at JJ hospital? I have never seen anybody after I left there. Matilda lives with me. She also works here. We love it here. The pay is much better and rosters are more comfortable. You should join us. You will like it here," Sheena enticed.

"I will certainly think about it."

"Let me know. I can pull some strings for you."

'Okay I must go. It was good to meet you. Bye for now."

"Bye"

Carmen hurried out hoping not to encounter anyone else. She had arranged to drop in at James' apartment after her appointment. On the way to James' apartment her mind was occupied with new plans. A new situation was evident now and she had to get prepared.

She was determined to be a great wife for James. She had to question him about the particular foods he liked and learn his Australian culinary favourites. Her mother had hammered into her that the only way to a man's heart was through his stomach. She remembered her own cooking sessions with her mother several years ago. This advice had to be heeded now. She would have to get more interested in life in Australia. That would please James very much. She wondered what the houses in Australia were like. She must read all about it at the library. Hopefully he may want to live in the bush. She could show kangaroos to the baby. She wondered how she would get a job in nursing there, would her qualifications be recognised and registerable, whether she would need more training. Were the any Indian nurses there? James would know. Whatever was required she was determined· to do. Her mind jabbered on, allowing her to take pride in her good fortune. How good is life?

Suddenly she recognised a heavily wrinkled smiling face. Yes, of course it was Marilyn's grandmother. Marilyn was a school friend who was now an air hostess.

"Hello Carmen. How are you?"

"I am good. How are you?"

"I am good by the grace of God."

"How is Marilyn?"

"She is always busy. I do not see much of her."

"Give her my regards when you see her next time," Carmen laughed.

"What are you doing here?"

"I just went to the hospital to see a nurse friend."

But Marilyn's grandmother didn't come down in the last shower. She had lived all these years with the sole objective of not being stupid. She deciphered that one does not usually see a friend at their place of work, particularly a nurse friend. You have a problem yourself dear or you want a job at the hospital, she deciphered in her mind. Nevertheless she decided that she would not probe on this matter further.

"How is Felicity? I have not seen her for a very long time."

"She's very good. Anyway I must go"

"One bit of advice before you go dear. Stay close with your family and friends. And avoid toxic people. And if you meet my Marilyn tell her that too."

"I will. Bye."

When she arrived at James' apartment she appeared manifestly elated. "I have some good news for you"

"Really what?" James just hoped to hear that she was not pregnant.

"You are soon to be a father. Congratulations."

"Oh, thank you. Did they tell you that?"

"I have just returned from the doctor at Breach Candy Hospital. The pregnancy test is definitely positive the doctor said."

"I think you should have the test repeated at another place also. So you can be absolutely sure."

Carmen saw the logic of his thinking, "Yes that's a very good idea. I will do that."

However he was already convinced that the die was cast.

They went down for lunch and she noticed that James was not his usual self. He was quiet and pensive and appetiteless. As was she. Perhaps the news was too sudden and unexpected and they needed time to let it sink in.

There was no sex on this day. The excuse provided by him was that he did not want to disturb her insides and the baby. That sounded logical to her although she was looking forward to an episode.

He asked her what her plans were now, hoping she would consider an abortion.

However, her decision was a very catholically substantiated no.

"I think we should get married before I actually begin to show. Don't you think? "

James was not prepared for this bombshell.

"Yes, yes."

Next she expected him to plan the baby's future with her.

"Do you think we should have the baby in Australia?"

"Yes, yes, definitely."

At this stage James really wanted to be left alone and have the time to plan his next move. He was totally obfuscated with the situation and realised what a dolt he had been. This was going to happen anyhow under the circumstances. Usually he was a very cautious lover. How did he let his caution to the wind this time? However it has happened now and he had to deal with it. But how?

He requested her to go home and rest as much as possible so the baby could gain hold at this early stage. She understood the logic of his concern and obliged by announcing that she would leave and promising to rest as much as possible. However she would see him again at work tomorrow.

"Yes", James assured her and planted his lips half-heartedly on her red lipstick imprinted lips.

When she left James' mind got to work. He absolutely did not want to father the child. But what can he do now under the circumstances? He cannot wait and let things roll. He decided to leave for home soon, like tonight.

He took a taxi to the airline offices at Churchgate and booked his flight to Sydney leaving at fifteen minutes to midnight. He was pleased that a seat was available for his escape. He went back to his apartment and packed hurriedly and called a taxi for eight o'clock. Luckily the apartment was prepaid and there would be no issues there.

The phone rang at precisely six o'clock. He knew it was Carmen. He decided not to answer. On her part Carmen thought he had gone out to celebrate his new position. She rang again at nine o'clock. This time he was not there to answer. Carmen had a ghoulish feeling that something was not right. She would wait till the morning and see him in the ward tomorrow.

She got into bed but sleep evaded her for a very long time. She had thoughts about the baby. It did not matter to her whether it was a boy or a girl. Dowries are not important for girls in Australia where marriages are decided on love. If it is a boy, he will definitely be a doctor just like James. With such pleasant thoughts sleep finally robbed her of her conscious state.

She woke up tired and hurried off to work. At work she felt soporific and was very decidedly taciturn. She kept her eyes open for James but alas he was nowhere to be seen. Something had happened. Did he get into trouble perhaps under the influence of alcohol?

Her abject condition was noted by some co-staff who were not aware of her romantic embroilments.

"Are you okay? You don't look well?"

"Did you eat something to upset your tummy?"

"I'm okay," Carmen responded to the various queries.

"No Carmen, you better go home. We can manage," the senior sister Mary Thandavan ordered.

"I'm okay," Carmen prevaricated, wishing not to miss on being on the lookout for James. At midday lunch time she rang James. There was no answer. Something was not right. Now she was really worried.

The other doctors did not seem to have noticed his absence. Essentially his position at the hospital was superfluous and his absence did not preclude any progress in their day's itinerary.

But Carmen was uneasy. There was nobody she could speak to in the hospital without arousing suspicion.

After work she went to his apartment at Breach Candy and it was locked. Now she was in a real panic. Something very bad had happened.

She could not go to the police without them interrogating her involvement and her own cause for concern. They may even find her a suspect if there was any mischief that they could not work out. Such is the nature of the police. If she was not pregnant she could have let things lie and just walk away. Where was James when she needed him most? What should she do?

James was in the air attending to his own thoughts. The flights had been delayed both in Bombay and Singapore. He was contemplating how they could have been so careless with the contraception? Sooner or later this would have happened under these circumstances. It was good while it lasted. Carmen was a nurse and should have known better. It was entirely her fault to lead him on. I only hope she fares okay.

As James' plane was approaching Kingsford Smith Airport in Sydney, James' thoughts now reverted to how he would get back to Newcastle. He would hire a car at the airport and drive back. He would inform his interrogators in the family and at the hospital that the Indian food did not agree with him and hence he was back earlier than expected.

Back in Newcastle at the hospital, he was quizzed by some for returning back sooner than they expected but there was no hesitancy to include him immediately on the on call roster. James had no objections. It would provide him some relief from his questioning conscience.

His thoughts about Carmen did not leave him soon. He tried hard to justify his own actions often blaming Carmen for the outcome. It was not his duty to tell her about contraception and remind her about the daily dosage. However he still felt uncomfortable for Carmen and often considered going back. But what excuse would he give her for running away? She would definitely never trust him again. What explanation would he have for his parents and the hospital? What would they think of him?

9

Apart from the doctor at the Breach Candy Hospital and James who knew about her current situation, Carmen was alone in her plight. No one else knew she was pregnant. Her mother Felicity and her brother Cecil were completely unaware that Carmen had had an affair with James. How best could she break the news to them now? She would tell her mother first. Cecil may be sympathetic but he pulled no weight with her mother. She decided to take it head on that evening after work and talk to her mother having guessed and prepared for her expected diction. Carmen was mentally preparing to leave town if required.

Later at home, noting that Cecil was not around, "Mum can I speak to you about something?" This was an unusual request from Carmen for Felicity.

"About what? You have not lost your job have you?" Felicity always attempted to pre-empt information on a disaster.

"No, something worse than that."

What can be worse than that? A police matter? Felicity wondered.

Felicity was all ears "What is bothering you?

"I'm pregnant"

For a second Felicity was speechless and looked at Carmen in disbelief. This cannot be true. You are pulling my leg. Not you, my daughter? Unwed? No way. However these things can happen after one misleading episode. She remembered times when her own uncle, Ernest had bothered her as a teenager. He often attempted to fondle her breasts just when they were just begging for recognition. He attempted to swipe his hands at her thigh juncture as if accidentally. However there was no coitus. But it could have happened. Felicity's mother was aware and had warned her to leave the room when he arrived. Uncle Ernest got the message and stopped visiting.

"Who is the father?"

"You don't know him? He is a doctor at the hospital."

Felicity surmised that can't be too bad. A doctor for a son in law. All her prayers had been eventually answered. She could walk around with her head held high and bear all the jealously in spite of her widowed condition. Her emotional humiliation would soon abate. May be God works in mysterious ways as the padre man usually says.

"Does he know? What did he say?"

"He has disappeared."

"What do you mean? A doctor can't just disappear."

"I feel he has gone back to his country I think."

"His country? Where is that?"

"Australia."

"What was he doing at JJ apart from getting you pregnant?"

Felicity soon realised that things were more complicated and may be difficult to sort out.

She wanted to know what led to all this and Carmen obliged her with all the major details. Felicity took consolation from the fact that she did not use contraception as forbidden by the church. At least she had got that bit right!

"This is God's punishment for me. What will everybody say about us? Do you know where you have put the family? Thank God your father is not alive. What are you going to do with the baby?" Felicity ruminated.

"I have thought about it and decided to keep the baby."

Under these circumstances Felicity felt the catholic rules could be flexible. Even priests with illegitimate outcomes in their affairs often resorted to abortion.

"I think you should have an abortion. We can find someone who could arrange. I know Laura's daughter had an abortion when she fell pregnant to Father Comen."

Carmen looked her mother in the eye and spoke directly, raising her voice," I will keep the baby. I will deal with it myself."

"Of course you will and Cecil and I really will really not suffer any consequences from your decision," Felicity retaliated.

Carmen had considered the situation privately and had thought of even moving out, even interstate if required although the thought of leaving her mother alone was not very comfortable.

She had never spoken to her mother in this manner before and began to feel guilty.

"I'm sorry mum. I didn't mean it that way."

"I don't think I will be able to face anyone at the bazaar anymore. I feel like hanging myself," Felicity acted it out to convey its full and entire meaning. And the consequences to every member of the family both alive and dead, of the unwed pregnancy to a foreigner were delineated, often in great detail as the ranting got deeper and more penetrating.

Carmen bore it all. She really had no feasible choice. She understood wherein her own fault lay. If only she had taken some birth control pills. But they were difficult to obtain as the family doctor was himself a strict catholic with nine children. She could not bear to listen to his homily and the associated leakage of such information to her holy mother.

When Cecil, her brother who was a year older than Carmen arrived home a while later, Felicity informed him of the news with her appropriate weightings and the requisite lachrymose accompaniments. Cecil was always an obligatory passive listener in his mother's interpretations of all matters. He had learnt from experience that Felicity had a propensity and tendency to alter the facts as necessary to aid her own point of view. Under such circumstances, her narrative ultimately turned the story into fiction. He had to talk to Carmen himself.

He asked Carmen if she would go for a walk with him at Chowpatty beach which she gladly accepted. A taxi was ordered and the driver delivered his passengers to Chowpatty beach.

"Tell me Carmen, I hear you have decided to keep the baby?"

"Yes Cecil. I have thought long and hard about it."

"It is entirely your decision as long as you fully understand all the consequences. And whatever your decision, I will support you."

"Thank you Cecil," Carmen knew she would have no problems with Cecil.

"You have a lot to know about men, Carmen."

"I took the short cut and burnt my fingers."

"All men want sex. To attain that they are polite and charming. These are essentially evasive qualities that conceal the truth. All women want security long term. To attain this they use sex."

"I know that. Papa used tell us that do you remember?"

"Yes. He would not be happy."

"I know. I am very sorry. I did love James. And I thought he loved me too," Carmen shed a tear.

"What has happened is in the past now. We have a chance to plan the future. But still we have no control."

She had heard all this before from papa, from Felicity, at church, at work and everywhere. But true love is never a logical phenomenon and therein lay the essence. People who have never been in love never understand it and there is no need to explain it to those who have. She had loved James.

"I have a feeling I will love your baby and I am sure mum will too when it arrives," James consoled.

Carmen smiled. She felt a bit better after this

conversation. She could almost visualise the baby with James' blue eyes and smile. She felt ready and would take them all on, if required. Cecil was a true brother.

As they were about to take a taxi back they recognised Erin, a friend of the family walking hurriedly toward them and waving with both hands. Erin was a school friend of Carmen and now a school teacher. She often came for an evening walk at Chowpatty. Her accompanying son, Basil, about four years of age seemed almost lost in this encounter. Meeting Erin was the last thing Carmen needed at this particular time.

"Hello Carmen. Hello Cecil. How are you?"

"Very good," They both choroused.

"And how is your mum?"

"She is very good," Carmen replied hoping not to provide any facial clues.

"How are you and Jake going?" Cecil inquired.

"We are well. We have a new puritan principal at the school. Insists on knee length uniforms for girls and hates kids listening to the devil's music."

"So what's new since we finished school there?" Carmen said.

Suddenly Basil darted off as fast as his legs could cooperate exclaiming, "I'm going home"

Erin with her teacherly screams threatened him with physical trauma which could emanate from the surrounds presently and later from her as well. The boy appeared unconcerned and carried on regardless. Cecil commanding his athletic skills which had not provided much help in his own school days chased him and soon the boy was derailed off the ground and carried back to his mother's arms. Erin thanked him profusely and begged their leave whilst still admonishing the young unconcerned Basil who had been through her such unfulfilled threats, many times before.

When they got home, Felicity had already planned a visit for Carmen and herself to see the local priest, Father Appollinaris Pereira. He was a tall cleric with a black framed spectacles and devoid of any hairy scalp cover and usually considered reverently sagacious although his basic duties involved only the church stock purchases at which he was profitably adept at outbidding his sellers.

Carmen was marched off to the interview. Father Pereira was delighted to see them both or so he expressed.

"We have a problem father," Felicity started.

Father Pereira only hoped this was not a request for money. Nevertheless he pre-empted, "How much do you need?"

"Not money Father," Felicity said.

He breathed a sigh of relief.

"What is it then Felicity?"

"Carmen is pregnant."

Father Pereira quickly ran through his mind which priest might be most likely this time. Not Comen again he hoped. Comen was a handsome Spanish priest with blue eyes and an athletic build who was a magnet for the local girls. His wand was powerful and apparently quite effective.

"Who is the father? Do we know?" He really didn't

think Carmen was promiscuous.

"An Australian doctor." Felicity added.

He breathed a sigh of relief, "Is he a Catholic?"

"He has had fled the country," Felicity added further.

"Did he leave an address behind?"

"No" Carmen intervened.

"That's what they do. We also have many Indian foreign doctors who come here and get proposal marriages, collect the dowry and flee back to their foreign white wives and children. There is nothing that can be done. It's always buyer beware," Father Pereira advised.

"He is white. And there is no dowry question," Carmen filled in.

"Well Carmen. These things happen. They are the work of the Almighty to try us. All we can do is pray."

Carmen's feathers were being ruffled, "Pray for what outcome father? Miscarriage?"

"No my dear. Remember God works in mysterious ways. We cannot work the mind of God. I will say a prayer for you."

"Thank you father. You will have to come and have a meal with us," Felicity offered.

"I would be delighted. I am usually free on Wednesdays."

"We will let you know," Carmen finished abruptly.

Father Apollinaris understood the young ones these days and preferred to ignore her tone. He knew that if the minds of the older parents are captured the young ones are then automatically reined in. He remembered a discussion with a senior cleric once who had informed him that once you win the minds of the elders, their moneys and children will invariably follow.

Both mother and daughter took leave and left, Carmen angrier than ever.

"Father is right. God has his own ways," Felicity said.

Carmen was at a loss to express herself further and bit her lower lip. She saw the mountain she was up against. Instinct, ignorance culture and tradition. James had once discussed with her about the guilt ridden Augustine of Hippo, son of a devout alcoholic mother and his vocative confessions letter addressed to god. The god who really was uninformed of Augustine's inner thoughts and his whereabouts! The god who helps those who help themselves. If you can help yourself what is the need for a god to help you? Carmen suddenly realised she was beginning to think.

Essentially the clerics were panjandrums who could only impress the females in the parish. Like Augustine of Hippo's father, most of the males in the parish did not succumb to their divine-authorised disciplinary Sunday orations and employed the set time to meet at the local cafe during the homily. It was easy to decipher that they attended Sunday church merely to escape the homily from their wives and mothers if they did not attend. 'You are setting a bad example for the children or what will the neighbours say about us?' An hour of one's life every week for a peace deal at home. Bargain.

Carmen attempted to sleep that night with thoughts of that bastard James, her mother's hysterics, Cecil's placidity and Father Apollinaris' conniving. She knew worse times were to follow when the baby would begin to show. For once she felt she wanted a boy. She would buy him a superman cape! She had read enough of those comics when Cecil brought them home regularly when they were at school. She really loved them then. With these thoughts, sleep finally had its way with her whist her mother snored away in the near vicinity.

The mornings usually portended normalcy apart from Felicity's expected catastrophe rants. The days paved way to weeks and months and the baby was making its presence known and Carmen was beginning to show. Word was getting around that Carmen had a problem. They all wanted to know 'Who is the father?' Every bachelor, married male, grandfather and cleric were subjected to suspicion at one time or another.

Many a child had his ear flipped at school when they enquired if it may not be a miracle.

Meanwhile at homes in the vicinity, discussions raged every day.

"I hope it's not you," Mary would say to John.

"Why me? I have six children already."

"Then why do you come home so late and drunk?"

"I go for a drink with my friends after I knock off at the bank."

"Is Carmen your friend?"

"I will knock your jaw in if you don't stop now. Right now."

"Why are you so upset if it's not you?"

And some jaws were indeed objectively manipulated requiring police and ambulance intervention.

Some even implored the possibility that Cecil may be the father. Who knows? Men will be men.

Her mother, Felicity took to very early morning bazaaring to avoid the goan questioning and was agoraphobic later in the day and night bemoaning her plight verbally and imploring the Almighty to take her away to join her husband. The Almighty of course never interfered in such human matters. It had more important things to do, that is to look for places to hide which were getting more and more scarce.

Carmen obtained leave from the hospital and stayed at home often seeking mental solace from being alone. She remembered James with hatred. She found a copy of *Gombrich* that he had presented her. She thought of burning it but something inside her would not allow, more for the value of its contents rather than her affection for James. Also she was uneasy about burning books. She always felt it was wrong. Only Hitler and the Catholic Church could do such things! She remembered particularly how *Gregor Mendel's* work on genetics was destroyed by his superiors in the monastery immediately after his death for fear of interfering with the church's teachings.

She spent a lot of time reading and in mental discussions with herself. James had advised her to learn how to think not what to think. This was a new horizon. Although she felt she hated him for what he had done to her, there were many things she learnt from him that she would not have encountered otherwise. No one would be able to understand that. It was solely her own experience only. She felt grateful inside. Maybe God works in mysterious ways!

Realising her impending predicament Carmen now sought refuge in books. She found solace in reading *Anthony De Mello*, a Jesuit priest who had published some books and she began to make some notes from his books. Her notes were very comprehensive. She noted that De Mello's books contained some valid elements of oriental wisdom in revealing the influence of Buddhist and Taoist spiritual currents and he eventually managed to achieve a progressive distancing from the essential contents of the Christian faith. In place of the revelation which has come in the person of Jesus Christ, De Mello substituted an intuition of god without form or image, to the point of speaking of god as a pure void. This radical negative theology she noted led to a denial that the Bible contains valid statements about god. She remembered that James had also talked similarly. De Mello mentioned that the words of Scripture only serve to lead a person to silence and to prevent people from following their own common sense. Hence religions, including Christianity, De Mello deciphered are one of the major obstacles to the discovery of truth. De Mello considered god as a cosmic reality, vague and omnipresent. He ignored the personal nature of god. He advised that belief or profession of faith whether in god or in Christ impedes one's personal access to truth that made us capable of growth. A capacity for the present, De

Mello stressed, was the secret to happiness because it saved us from the hurts of the past and the tyranny of a fearful future. Ruminating on the past gives us depression and ruminating about the future gives us anxiety. We lose happiness when we make it dependent on anyone or anything else. The secret to happiness is that it lies within us by our ability to find satisfaction within ourselves. He also stressed that we must be open to unlearning everything we have ever known in life if we are going to be able to grow from one place to another. The past is to be dropped because it is past. Beliefs trap us into close-minded positions. We have to stop seeking perfection. No, James would not agree with that. He would seek perfection. Religion, De Mello pointed out is not necessarily connected with spirituality. Spirituality for De Mello is the ability to live whole and happy in the now, expecting nothing, demanding nothing, grasping nothing and so becoming open to all things. De Mello claimed that, one of the biggest obstacles to truth is religion. She could easily agree with all that. James had taught her how to think. However James had gone even further and denied the very existence of a god.

De Mello mentioned that in their god-driven searches, mystics roam far afield from the safety of institutional pronouncements, a roaming often interpreted from the outside as a kind of withdrawal from responsibilities to the world. Prayer as the inner fire makes people withdraw from human relations and make them lose their appetite for life. Equipped with these notes she resolved she could seek her own truth. She was not aware that irrespective, religion has a propensity to target the lonely and depressed and the love forlorn! Could she be a sitting duck herself?

10

As he tried to seek his life back at the Royal Newcastle Hospital, the memory of Carmen haunted him. Was that the right thing and moral thing to do? Should he not have known better and not have got involved or used some form of contraception? He could have used condoms but he liked the feeling of skin on skin. Besides he did not like the interruption of having to stop, to put it on. Should he go back to her? What would she say? Would she ever trust him again after what he did? Could he offer to marry her now? What would his own mother and father and other colleagues say? Such thoughts refused to leave him alone. Too many complications he thought. He wondered how Carmen might be managing. There was no way of knowing. Such questions sought to occupy his mind and interfere with his sleep and functioning for a long time. What kind of person would desert a girl he made pregnant? Was it because she was Indian? Hardly. He was well past that. Then what was it? Yes it was the racism in his family and friends. They may not accept her. And he suffered mentally. Often, when not on call he would go to a pub all by himself and think and think and think. Time however heals and his guilt eventually retracted very slowly.

He dated some of the nurses at the hospital but his heart just refused to co-operate.

In time he noticed Freida Bryne, a research scientist at the hospital was beginning to pull his heart strings and he was beginning to feel he was ready for more serious romance outcomes. Freida was amply gifted anatomically and was igniting his long dormant hormones. She had shoulder length dark blonde hair and deeply set blue eyes that stared right into a face and a smile that reminded him very much of *Suzi Quatro*. Her talking voice had a soprano quality with a bright timbre. Not definitely a rock and roll voice but definitely a rock and roll body which visually delighted him. He could imagine her singing, *"Tear me apart if you want to win my heart."* He also recognised that her body fragrance had notes of cat urine as in a Sauvignon Blanc, a wine which he liked. This may be a quasi-*Marcel Proust* phenomenon when a person's smell reminds you of a wine?

Freida did notice that she was the object of his desires and was determined to take advantage of his vulnerability. Her own current romantic adventure was waning.

One Friday evening when he found her alone he took his chances and asked her to join him for a drink at the Great Hunter Hotel which she accepted. They arranged to meet that evening and as usual James arrived there first. He went in and was escorted to a table by the window. He ordered a glass of Sauvignon Blanc before she arrived which was just a few minutes later.

She was wearing navy blue jeans and a pink silk chiffon blouse which exposed some of her cleavage. As he moved his gaze around her blouse, the lustre in the cloth appeared to change colour. He wondered what other surprises lay hidden underneath. He would wait to find out. Only time will tell. He just hoped that the Stanford marshmallow experiment was true for adults also and his waiting would reward him.

She sat opposite him. She noticed he had a habit of rolling his tongue which she interpreted as a nervous disposition perhaps related to his first date with her.

To ease his perceived discomfort she inquired, "Have you been waiting long?"

"No. I just got in a few minutes ago. Tell me what will you have?"

"A chardonnay will do me fine," she replied

He went to the bar and got her a glass of chardonnay.

When he returned Freida said, "It was nice of you to ask me for a drink."

"No problem. I was waiting a long time for the moment. It was nice of you to accept."

"I had noticed you for some time myself. I thought you'd never ask. Do you come here often?" Freida inquired.

"I do. I find the food is good here. Just in case you are hungry"

"Yes. I will accept that offer too."

"What will you have?"

"I prefer to finish this wine first."

"Of course," James felt he may have some luck in this venture.

"So do you like your job?"

"Very much so," James responded rolling his tongue again.

"I could easily guess that," Frieda added, "I have been watching you clandestinely."

Next they talked about his family. Freida had not realised that Rodney, the ear, nose throat surgeon was his father. He informed her that he did his initial training at the Royal Newcastle Hospital with a stint at the Royal Prince Alfred in Sydney and St Vincent's Hospital in Melbourne. Later he trained himself under the National Health System at Leeds in England for two years.

"What do you mean you trained yourself?" she asked.

"Basically there was no supervision. You read an operation, did one and taught one. I never saw some of the consultants at all."

"I would hate that if I were a patient. How did the patients feel about that?"

"Basically, the non-affording had no choice."

"Were there private hospitals and private insurance?"

"Yes. That's where the consultants spent their time."

"I see."

She filled him in with her family information next. She was from Sydney, Asquith to be precise. She informed him that she had a PhD from Sydney University, about her interest in comparative cleft lip and palate genetics, her current involvement with cats and the various papers she had already written along with the joys, plights and the fierce competition for those seeking funds for research and information regarding the writing of research proposals.

"Currently my research is centred on cat cleft lip and palate. I have a joint grant from Boston University in the United States and the Feline Health Research Fund."

"That's interesting. I am planning to eventually restrict my work to cleft palate and lip surgery if there is enough such work in Newcastle."

"You can do vet work." Freida joked.

"No, not my cup of tea. I don't like uncommunicative patients or those ungrateful ones that bite."

"I see your point. Like humans, cleft palate is usually an inherited congenital disorder in cats. There is a breed predilection. It's more likely to occur in purebred cats and is commonly found in Norwegian forest cats, spotted ocicats, Persians, ragdolls, savannahs, and Siamese breeds. It occurs in female cats more often than males."

"I suppose certain chemical agents can also contribute," James interrupted with his knowledge of the human factors.

"Of course. Cleft palates can also be caused by exposure of pregnant female cats to teratogenic chemicals. These chemicals include griseofulvicin and excessive vitamin A and vitamin D. In these cases, the kittens may be born with cleft palates."

"Do you have much to do with dogs?" James inquired.

"No. Not at work. But I am interested in comparative biology particularly genetics. It is also common in dogs particularly purebred brachycephalic breeds. You know the ones with short noses like Bulldogs, Boston terriers, Pekinese. Again nutritional deficiencies, viruses and toxins during the bitch's pregnancy increase the risk," Freida replied.

"Perhaps if you did more research on Boston terriers, then Boston University may increase you grant," James said.

"Sorry, that's not how it works mate."

"Just joking."

"I believe a long time ago a Bostonian man crossed a white English terrier with French bulldogs to produce the Boston terrier. Did you know Boston University has a Boston Terrier for its mascot?"

"I did not know that."

James was now able to decipher why she always had the sauvignon blanc note in her aroma reminding him of the cat urine note in the wine.

"Okay I think I know something about you now. Now that we have ruled out that you are not aligned with the mafia, what do you want to eat? Here is the menu," James pushed the menu on the table towards her.

She had a quick look, "I could do with a pizza. I will take the Margherita."

"The pizzas are good here. I might take the meatlovers one. More wine?"

"Why not?" she responded.

He trotted off to the bar and ordered and paid. He came back with the wines and placed them on the table.

"Just a bit more about yourself. Are you currently romantically involved?" James asked.

"I have a decaying relationship with Arthur who is the professor of molecular genetics at Sydney University. Arthur is already married and promised me he would get a divorce which has not eventuated yet and I sense he has no real intentions. So I am amenable to other romantic offers."

James' alarms went off. Stop, stop. Hold it James. Don't jump. You have burnt your fingers once that have not healed completely yet and obviously do need grafting but is this donor suitable? Wait.

Freida had a very saline sense of humour which was amusing and offensive at times particularly when she referred to the professor. She described him as being a Neanderthal with simian features and referred to him as "Simo".

James was selfishly pleased with her response towards the professor.

Lighter conversation followed and the waiter arrived with the pizzas and plates. They decided to share the pizzas.

James was grateful she was not a vegetarian or vegan or any other form of dietary proletarian. He could not cope with that. He had met some women who could spend an entire evening's dinner date just pulling out the peas or bacon or garlic out of the meal on to the side of the plate, in the very meal they had ordered for themselves with all the ingredients adequately mentioned in the menu listing.

After the meal James inquired "What are you doing this evening?"

"Nothing that can't wait. Would you want to come over to my place in Mayfield? I have some nice brandy which I am willing to share with you."

Exactly just what James wanted to hear, "That sounds like a good idea"

"Okay here's my address and telephone number in case you need to be rescued without police intervention." She wrote her address on a piece of paper and handed it to him.

James perused the paper, "I know where that is."

They walked out with her holding on to his arm and he escorted her to her car which was parked in the library cark park a few metres away.

"See you soon," she retorted as she drove off in her Honda Civic.

"Yeah," he replied as he waved her off.

On the way to her apartment, James stopped at a bottle shop and picked a Moet. He also got some orchids from the florist next door. He thought that she might appreciate that.

On arrival at her apartment he gifted her with his purchases.

She thanked him with a very protracted kiss.

The apartment had a fragrance of vanilla with caramelised marshmallow which James was able to ascribe to the wax candle sitting on the coffee table. She appeared to love wax candles just like Janet. Frieda had a modest two bedroom apartment with minimal furniture to include two armchair sofas, an ottoman and a circular coffee table in the lounge on which also nested a copy of *Caravaggio The Complete Works* by *Sebastian Schutze*.

"I didn't know you like *Caravaggio*," he asked as he scanned the copy.

"Oh, I just love his work," she replied.

"His drama is too intense for me and he spills all over the picture."

"I just love that. And I am not going to stop now."

"Okay, I am not even going to try to stop you."

"Will you have some brandy?" she asked.

"Yes. Definitely. Thank you."

"Okay give me a few ticks," she walked abruptly to the kitchen.

She came back with a bottle of St Agnes XO Grand Reserve brandy and two brandy glasses.

"I just love this. It has a lovely caramel toffee flavour," she commented.

She poured both glasses.

"Keep helping yourself," she said.

"We also have a bottle of Moet to finish," he added.

"We have a young evening on our side," she replied.

"Indeed we do."

The conversation drifted towards the hospital and the various mutually known staff and their humorous peculiarities.

"Do you know Viola 'crash helmet'?" she asked

"Who doesn't? It's a pity she was not wearing her helmet when she was being delivered. That may have saved her from her congenital brain fog."

"I agree. Apparently when she rides her bike she insists that two vehicles have the same right to occupy the same portion of the road at the same time. According to her, all vehicles are created equal and have the same rights."

The   booze   flowed   and   the   conversation

deteriorated.

"You might as well stay tonight. I am not happy to see you driving back after all that alcohol. After all, you are considered the sane pillars of our society and rash behaviour on your part is not acceptable. You can sleep in my bed provided you are not too naughty."

It was not necessary to go through the, 'what will the neighbours say' routine in their current circumstance.

Together they undressed and got into bed with minimal fuss.

Before long their sexual urges took control of their bodies. It did not take him long to be inside her and having discharged his contents he drifted off to asleep. She did not orgasm although she felt she was close. She could have faked it as she regularly did with Simo. She thought of *Meg Ryan* in *When Harry met Sally*. At least it was a start. Next time she hoped they would not drink as much.

He woke up early and was wondering about her contraception. He did not want to be caught in his previous plight again although he felt he could handle it much better now.

His thoughts drifted to Carmen. What a bastard he had been? He wondered how she might be managing the shame and scandal in her community. Nevertheless he had shifted to a different life now and he must not let these thought bother him.

Just then Freida opened her eyes and recognised

him.

'Oh are you still here? Don't you have work to do?"

"Yes I do. Shall we start?"

"Give me a second to empty my bladder and I will be back. Don't move. I've got you covered," She threw the sheets over him to aid her pun.

"Go ahead. Make my day," he responded.

It was Saturday. He had hospital rounds to do this morning. The residents would be waiting for him. He rang his registrar from the lounge and told him to go ahead as he was delayed elsewhere.

When he returned she was already in bed and denuded of all underwear.

"Freida, you know about contraception, don't you?"

"It's been taken care of."

He jumped into bed and into another round of sexual gymnastics. This time they both orgasmed together. It was perfect he thought. Such timing had never happened to him before. This time it was him thinking, she could be faking a *Meg Ryan*.

Nonetheless she clearly was his favourite thus far. Should he look any further if this was working? A bird in hand literally? Should he work on marriage here, he thought. After all he was getting on in years, as his mother reminded him every time he visited her. Freida would get on well with his mother and Janet. And he loved her cat urine odour which literally turned him on. What more? He did not know how she stood on thinking about life and its complexities. May be he needed to explore that a bit further.

As they lay there, enumerating their common invidious personalities at work, he remembered that he had to go to the hospital. He got out of bed and showered and dressed. He took leave of Freida after asking her to join him for lunch at Fanny's bar at noon. On his way to the hospital he pondered on the propitious romantic turn his life may take from now on. However he resolved that he may need to guide Freida in abstaining from small talk which usually did irritate him considerably. He remembered the lithe Yorkshire girl, Olivia who never could stop her verbal literation even on noticing that he was not listening. Under the circumstances he was prepared to consider that last night was an exigent preliminary testing situation but such a recurrence must be precluded in the future. He felt he had work to do. Would Freida co-operate and comply?

11

He arrived at the hospital as his team was seeing the last patient. After excusing himself for his delayed appearance, he quickly acquainted himself with the progress of the patients from the registrar, Matt and was pleased with the post-operative outcomes.

"How is the man we did with the mandible reconstruction?"

"He's fine. The wound looks good. Would you like to see him?"

"Yes."

The procession did an about turn and went toward the man in bed nine.

The nurse was putting the finishing touches on his bandages.

"Hold on nurse, Dr Regan wants to see the wound," Matt interrupted her.

The nurse reversed her movements and undid the bandage. James examined the wound and was pleased with the results and requested the nurse to finish after apologising for the excess work he had subjected her too. The nurse, as usual put on a "no problem" smile although within her, her thoughts were otherwise.

"Did you check the donor leg?" James inquired.

"Yes, that's fine too," Matt completed.

"Okay I think that's it for the moment. Right Matt?"

"Yes," Matt replied.

"How is your exam preparation coming up Matt?"

"Getting there."

"How are you going Mohan?" He asked the resident.

"I am sitting the primary in April next year in Melbourne"

"What about you Pete?" He asked the other resident.

"Me too"

They had a new intern, Reginald. He was embarrassingly smudged with facial freckles and had a minimal threshold for smiling. He had realised early that it was one the job requirements, irrespective of inner contradicting concerns.

"What about you Reggie? Are these guys treating you well?"

"Very good."

"Mohan and Pete, do you guys know how to write a medical journal paper?"

"Nobody teaches that," Mohan replied.

"I want you two and if you wish Reggie, to come to my office in about a quarter hour and we will talk about it."

"Can I come too?" Matt inquired.

"Of course you can."

"Sorry you may need to excuse me, they want me in the ward after I finish here," Reginald said.

"Yes of course, but you can join us later if you wish," James replied.

James then proceeded to his office in the old building. In between the two buildings he gazed at the sky above and burst into a fit of sneezing. He surmised the weather was promising of a nice day ahead. He was looking forward to meeting Freida for lunch. He busied himself in his office with some pending paperwork till the residents arrived.

When they arrived James requested them to find a chair and sit down. When they were all settled, "First of all in any of our scientific writing you must remember that you are writing for doctors who are guided only by facts and logic, not by emotion," James started.

"Emotion is for novels only, right?" Pete understood.

"Yes. If you ever use emotion in a scientific paper to persuade a reader you will immediately lose your credibility. Aristotle called it pathos. It is okay in other literature but not in science. You need to know how you, as an author can make a connection between your mind and in the mind of the reader about a specific topic, for a specific purpose and a specific occasion. At first you need to select a Central Research Question, CRQ for short that is based on what you think is new, that you can offer with your own twist with the available literature for evidence. For that you must know what is already out there.

"Good point," Pete commented.

"There are five steps you need to follow - Invention, Research, Drafting, Revising and Editing," James enumerated with the rolling of his tongue for punctuation. He had written several papers himself and was well suited to deliver this mini-talk.

"Wait, I need to make notes on this. Can you please say those steps again?" Mohan requested as he pulled his notebook out of his pocket.

"Hold on. I need to also," Pete added.

James repeated the steps slowly allowing them time to write.

"So what do you exactly mean by invention? Surely you don't mean we have to invent something," Matt was making notes too.

"No no. I mean thinking carefully, thoughtfully, and systematically about a project before undertaking it provides you with opportunities for reflection, preliminary planning, and effective time management. As much as possible make sure your question is not a yes-no question. Also avoid simple fact-based questions."

"Do you have any strategies for the CRQ?" Matt asked.

"No special strategies. Ask yourself why the question is important or why it matters. Who would be affected by the results of exploring the CRQ? Ask why this question should be explored right now. Think about what other questions a CRQ can make you think about. Does that make sense?"

They nodded.

Next let's talk about drafting."

"Isn't the next step Research?" Matt interrupted after he looked at his notebook.

"Yes I want to save that for a bit later. That's a bit complicated."

"Okay."

"Before you start drafting the article begin by introducing your article to the readers.

This usually happens in the first paragraph or in the first few paragraphs. Include a one or two sentence description of what will be demonstrated or what will happen in the larger piece of writing. Paragraphs help through the process of reading your article. Each paragraph should focus just on one main idea. A topic sentence is the first sentence in a paragraph and it generally introduces what the paragraph is going to be about. And finally in the conclusions alert the reader to the most important insights in the article. And give the reader some sense of why this insight is important. Okay so far?"

"I wish they taught us this in the English subject at school. All they stressed was 'show and tell' which I think nobody really understood anyhow," Pete admitted.

"Let's talk a bit about revision now. Is that okay?"

They all nodded again. This is getting interesting they all thought. Writing research papers is not easy.

"Revision can produce global changes that affect the whole of the article. It can shift perspectives, cause reconsideration of beginnings and endings, introduce new structures and orders, create a new approach to the subject, provide the inclusion of new sources and novel organization or structure. Can you understand how this can happen?"

They nodded.

"The draft will tell you if have achieved your goals for the project. Research or references can be used as evidence or to provide background information. You may need to spend long hours at the library for this and this can be great fun. In fact sometimes this puts me in 'flow'. Do you know what flow is?"

"Yes. Flow is when you become fully immersed and engrossed in an activity and lose any sense of time," Pete knew.

"Yes, that's right," James said.

"Very interesting," Matt interrupted.

"In References, there are two sources. Primary sources are sources that are the thing itself while the secondary sources are articles written about the primary source. Secondary sources are written by observers who interpret or analyse primary sources. So secondary sources can be used to see what others have discussed or get their opinions. Always check if the sources are credible, authoritative and peer reviewed. And as usual always check for potential bias. Do you get that?"

They nodded again.

"You must also learn how to summarise every source you read as to its thesis statement, main point and the purpose. We can leave that topic for discussion on another day if you wish."

"I am sure we'd all love that," Matt said

"And finally remember all research is always incomplete. Your article is not the final say on the subject just like what I have said thus far is not the last word on this subject. You will discover more as you read further. I think you have had enough from me. I should stop now." The lunch with Freida bells were also ringing for James.

"That was very good Dr Regan," Matt complimented," I'm glad I joined in."

"Yes really very good," Mohan and Pete chorused.

"Dr. Regan I have a personal question for you," Matt said.

Oh no this will definitely involve my bachelorhood he thought. Nevertheless he was ready.

"Yes what is it?"

"You seem to know a lot. How come?" Matt wanted to know.

"Usually Matt I would rather spend my time in a book. I am not fascinated by small talk and have saved a lot of time by avoiding it. Does that help?"

They all nodded again.

"Go shout that on the mountains," James laughed as they found their way out.

James was relatively rather pleased with himself after this episode with the residents.

At lunch time he drove to Fannys where Freida was already waiting inside at the same table as last time. She had already ordered a Sauvignon Blanc for him and a Chardonnay for herself and placed them on the table.

"I ordered for you. I thought it would save time considering the plans I have for you today. How are your patients doing? I hope as well as you, last night."

'No, not as good as that," he joked.

She smiled.

"Have you had a look at the menu?" he inquired.

"I feel like some fish today. I am going to settle for fish and chips. What about you?"

"Potatoes make me fart. I will have a burger," James replied.

"My turn to pay today," she got up to order.

"I am not going to be hard hearted and deprive you the privilege."

"Thank you. That settles that. I like men who do not argue. I think I am beginning to like you."

"That makes the two of us liking me," he joked.

She went off to order and pay. She returned in a short while, "You have not asked about my plans for you later."

"I'm sure you have no sadistic tendencies."

"Sadistic, what made you think of that?"

"I want to know if you will hurt me. I don't like planned pain."

"I would never hurt you or anyone for that matter, not physically anyhow."

"What about emotionally?"

"Emotionally yes, if you don't comply, as Simo is soon to find out."

That was some cheerful news for him.

"So what is your plan? I am curious to know."

"You will like my plan if you believe life is for living. Whether you use it or not, it just keeps on going."

"I like that. I think I will like your plan."

"To me if you enjoy what you do, money is not a bother."

"Are you going to be philosophical today?"

The waiter arrived with their meals and the conversation was suspended as they eyed the food. Both of them now attended to their hunger. After sometime James inquired, "How is the fish and chips?"

"Okay. And how is your burger?"

"Good, I like the mayonnaise sauce they use here. It has a touch of balsamic."

"Take some chips from me if you wish. I am not going to finish them all."

"Okay, but you have been warned of possible consequences."

"It's okay, I am getting used to your snoring and farting. I have already factored that in about you."

He forced a smile and took a chip from her plate.
He knew he liked her.

"What would you say if we drove to the vineyards today and spent the night there?"

"Don't you have to book?"

"All done. We should leave soon."

"Can I collect some clothes?"

"You will not need any clothes."

He knew what she meant. At least he thought he knew what she meant.

When they finished they drove to her apartment in their separate cars. From there, they left for the vineyards in his Series 2 E type convertible Jaguar. They were also equipped with minimal food and drink amenities.

On the way up, as he was driving he remembered he did not have any spare underwear.

"Hey, I have no spare underwear," he shouted with a rolled tongue. He had to raise his voice to be heard.

"Fine, you can borrow mine, but for a fee of a dollar a minute," she laughed back.

"That's expensive."

"Elementary economics Dr. Watson, if something is expensive, learn to do without it."

"I suppose that was your plan anyhow, Miss Sherlock Holmes."

"Aye, now you are beginning to understand the real Arthur Conan Doyle."

"Are you a fan of Sir Arthur?" James inquired.

"Not particularly. It was something I read in school."

"I noted you like philosophy," James commented.

"Up to a point when I am sort of inebriate and there is nothing else to do," she replied.

"I remember reading *Nietzche's Thus spake Zarathrustra*, a long time ago where he spoke of humans evolving eventually into superhuman beings. I think he called such beings *Ubermensch* or something like that. Nice thought. But this obviously is not to happen in my life time"

"Who is Zarathrustra?" Freida inquired.

"You may know him as *Zoroaster*. Zoroaster is the first guy to distinguish between good and evil. He founded Zoroastrianism in Persia, which is modern day Iran. Zoroastrianism is apparently the oldest religion. Incidentally to me all religions are a form of collective madness with disoriented reality which provides us enough strength to endure the misfortunes of others." These were Carmen's words, he remembered.

"That's interesting. We had a priest in our parish at Chatswood who always thanked God for saving us from a disaster somewhere else. He was always waiting for a catastrophe to happen elsewhere to claim how our own good God had saved us," Freida went on.

"Chatswood is becoming busy these days isn't it?" James asked.

"Very. My dad, Frederick was the Commonwealth Bank manager at Chatswood and he has noticed a vast change. Even my mother, Grace who was a senior claims consultant with GIO Insurance in the Workers Compensation Department mentioned that Chatswood is getting to be different now. You must meet them sometime soon."

'I'd love to," he responded.

"Perhaps next weekend. Can you manage?"

"I can arrange that."

"My dad, he almost hears nothing without his hearing aids and with them, only sometimes. He rarely wears them at home. But I must warn you about my mother, she is paranoidal with conspiratorial thinking and has a tendency to catastrophise as preparation for an actual catastrophe. I remember the endless arguments I used to have with her when I wanted to go out at night. She was morbidly fearful of me being raped by drunks. Nevertheless, I went out, never got raped but had her sitting up till two o'clock sometimes. I thought her job in insurance would help her understand that catastrophes and disasters are a fact of life."

"You are lucky you have such parents. My mother kept awake for Janet, my sister too. But not for me."

"Hey you watch out. There are some wild women out there willing to rape men."

"Come and get me," he laughed loudly.

"Coming."

"Incidentally Freida, what religion do you believe in?"

"I am a very very lapsed catholic. I noticed early in my life that nobody speaks the truth in religion least of all the priests, all being trained liars. They know only how to make better excuses for god. What about you? What are your beliefs?"

"Well, I don't believe in angels and holy spirits or Krishna or Zeus or Jupiter type of stuff."

"Point taken. I think we may be sitting on the same tree."

"Or on different branches perhaps."

"Yes, but remember the higher you go, the branches

get more fragile."

"And finally break or disappear," James tried to finish.

"To me, there are only two ways of living, the life you desire and the life you are born to. Sometimes these lives can be the same. Sometimes we try to make them the same."

"I like that," James complimented her.

"I like talking to you. You have some interesting things to say and also do."

"Thank you," he responded.

They were still some distance to cover to get to Pokolbin in the Hunter Valley. The car loved the unpaved roads which was a credit to British engineering and a saviour of their own spines!

12

It was continuing to be a very hot day. The clouds were not going to risk their life expectancy and had decided to take a day off from their usual annual sick leave quota. The cicadas however had other plans and had their mating orchestra going on in full swing. They would rather go for a species survival as was the functional trait amongst their lot.

As they were approaching Pokolbin, the speed of James' driving and the retracted sunroof was causing Freida's hair to blow and provide her with a very pleasant sensation. She looked beautiful he thought, as he glanced at her sideways. He was pleased with his unexpected good fortune.

"Oh how I love the wind in my hair as we drive," she shouted.

"Freida my dear, the first thing to remember is that there is no wind. What you are talking about is perhaps a relative wind, if you must insist in calling it wind. Don't you think?" James shouted back as if he was just plodding for an argument.

"Should I say breeze then?"

"I don't think breeze can ruffle your hair."

"What about draught or slipstream?"

"Slipstream is the air that's behind a fast moving car. You will need to be flying behind the car to catch the slipstream like birds flying in V formation," James shouted.

"What about blast then?

"If there is no movement of air how can it be a blast?"

"Okay one thing I agree with you is there is no wind." Freida conceded.

"Settled. Loser to pay for the damages."

"Agreed. In cash or kind?" Freida asked.

"Kind," James said

"Okay just be kind to me."

"I promise."

On arrival at Number Sixty Four at Pokolbin they parked the car in a dirt car space in front and presented themselves to the unmanned reception desk which had a fan going with no human to appease. Their arrival appeared to disturb the daily sleep routine of the Labrador retriever who was forced to elicit a few tenor barks as per his job description requirements. A gentleman who appeared to be in his early thirties appeared from behind the curtain and greeted them and introduced himself as Matt. He then apologised for not being at the desk and for the hot weather and for Pokolbin being so far away from Newcastle. When he realised he was running out of events and excuses, he pulled out his book and inquired of their identities.

"I have a booking in the name of Bryne," Freida said.

"Indeed you do. I have you for one night. You are at Le Cabanon villa. Here are the keys."

"Thank you. How do we get there?" Freida inquired.

"Just follow the directions. It is easy. There is some milk and coffee and wine in your villa. We have a café and restaurant on the premises. Ring me if you need anything. There are some leaflets there if you want to be adventurous," he said pointing towards the wall mounted leaflet holder on his left.

"Have a nice stay," he finished.

"Thank you," James nodded.

James and Freida watched the man as he disappeared again behind the curtain to rehearse for his next show. They collected a few leaflets.

The villa was sufficiently secluded and nestled near a dam amongst bushland. The ambience was most relaxing. Freida unpacked as James perused the leaflets. He had no unpacking to do.

"This is a great place. How did you come to know about it?" James inquired.

"My parents have stayed here before and they absolutely liked it."

"I would really like to meet them and congratulate them on this choice."

"On the weekend, we have agreed"

"Yes of course," James remembered.

After they had settled in, they decided to explore the surroundings. They particularly admired the Brokenback Range backdrop. They were both usurped with the natural beauty of the place and the friendly animals around including the pigs and goats which possibly were conditionally sacrificial pets. The wombats and kangaroos roamed around freely possibly fully aware of their own protection rights.

Watching the animals caused James to ponder.

"Penny for your thoughts" Freida laughed.

"I was just thinking do you know that the human

mind is the only one to reflect on its own nature and development. Our minds are unsurpassed in flexibility, imagination, creativity, and narrative ability, but they are also subject to distortions and biases as well as the potential for highly impairing mental disturbances," James began.

Fiona loved the comparative stuff, "The core difference between human brains and those of primates is not sheer size but the number of neurons in the cortex and the massive, high-speed interconnections across brain regions. Great apes have highly developed episodic skills, the ability to remember. These are found in other mammals, too. We humans are characterized by mimetic skills, involving imitation, gesturing, and other means of forging social bonds and cooperation."

"Yes, that's how we invented religions and its rituals to unite and cooperate," James added.

"And fight other religions too," Fiona laughed.

"Genes from our genetic heritage, which may have been quite adaptive during the cave segment of our evolutionary history, are no longer adaptive given the current environments we live in and thus cause our disordered functioning," James completed.

"It's great to be human isn't it?" Fiona responded. Thoughts now crossed her own imaginative and creative mind. She thought to herself that both she and James tend to go for the same topics. I am definitely going to make you mine James Regan, she thought. She looked him directly and a smile appeared on her face which James interpreted in his favour and mirrored one himself.

After a while Freida and James were tired of the sun stalking them and they decided to vamoose into the villa for a cuddle. The cuddle soon got complicated and other stand by anatomical machinery was appropriately recruited.

On completion of their urges, they both fell asleep. And woke up just in time for dinner. James who was always pragmatic chose a nearby restaurant to allay their hunger. The meal conversation revolved about families. His great grandfather had migrated to Australia from Limerick in Munster province in Ireland. Her great grandfather was also Irish from Cork in the same province. Armed with this information both of them decided to visit Munster next year together and explore their heritage.

"That sounds like a great idea," she agreed.

"As I told you before, great ideas run in my family."

The exact times and leave at the hospital needed to be organised.

"We shall work it out," James assured.

On the way back they stopped at a vineyard bottle shop for some wine to condition the remnant evening. Three bottles of Moet should suffice he thought.

Back at the villa, he opened a bottle and poured two glasses, offering Freida one.

After a few sips, Freida exhibited her salacious desires profusely by dancing a "can can" in her underwear to no music. James was impressed and joined her in some vacuous movements of his own. Finally she stopped and took her underwear off and threw it at James.

"How's that," he responded after catching her underwear and throwing it in the air.

"Your turn to bat now. Can you fix me with a sixer?" she replied

"Only if you throw me a *doosra*."

"What is a doosra?"

"Doosra really means "second" in hindi. In cricket it is an off-spin ball that swings the other way, confusing the batsman. So here's your chance to make me come on."

"Whatever. If cricket is your game, you will meet your match next weekend in my father. But please I implore you, don't start him," she warned.

"I promise."

The bed pitch was soft without much bounce and ideal. She went on top of him to continue the game and she did throw him a very favourable doosra. She did get a sixer, he thought. He felt lucky he found her. They both drifted off to sleep soon after.

When he woke up he heard the sulphur crested cockatoos shrieking outside protesting that their heavenly father had deserted them and they had to purloin food. His thoughts reared again. Was this real? Could Freida be the one for him? He liked her and her humour and her down to earth attitude so far. He especially liked her genitalcrian proclivities. After all, that would be a great help at the end of a long day of surgery. Also she appeared to be an evidence based logical person. Again he thought, should he ask her to marry him? He was getting on in years. What if she was just having a fling with him? So far his attempts at winning her had been hortatory, he thought. But then he really didn't know what was on her mind. The best way of finding was to ask her directly. What better way then asking her to marry him. So he resolved to ask when she woke up. Was that a good idea? Is it not too soon? It had only been days since he had met her. But she was exactly what he wanted and tomorrow might be another day. No, he should wait for a better time and perhaps place.

She opened her eyes a bit later with an accompanying smile.

"I will have to ring mum and tell her we are coming on the weekend," she remembered.

"So what plans do you have for this morning?" he wanted to know.

"I thought we could visit some vineyards if it's okay with you."

"Okay. That's fine. No cricket this morning. Let's move."

She went to the bathroom and in the meantime he for searched for the map of the vineyards that he had noted on the table when they initially arrived. He scanned the closest vineyards to where they were and noted them down. By the time she was finished he had it all planned and took himself to the bathroom.

The clouds were still adjusting their presence around the sun in the sky before they got started.

"We can breakfast at the first winery with their wine."

"Brilliant," she responded.

They breakfasted at Edgefall winery with the usual

bacon, eggs and toast routine.

During breakfast both of them were relatively taciturn, each pregnant with their own thoughts. They went to the cellar for the tasting and picked some chardonnay and merlot to take home.

The next winery they went to was Doverclift. The vineyard was spread over about forty acres with very pleasant and peaceful views. In spite of the absence of any evidence of rain, the odour emanating from the drying grass was pleasant like petrichor. There was some music being played. They picked some chardonnay and shiraz from the cellar.

Before long it was time for lunch and a light lunch of chicken burgers it was. During lunch James informed her that he had read that Pokolbin was the name used by the aboriginal people to mean 'a very hot place'. The other argument was provided by the early Hungarians to mean 'in the hell' in Hungarian. He informed her that shiraz and sémillon were the most popular wine varieties, but cabernet sauvignon, chardonnay, and pinot noir plantings could also be found throughout the surrounding countryside.

"Sorry James, my knowledge in these matters is very limited but I am willing to learn."

"I like that attitude Freida."

They went back to Le Cabanon and collected their belongings and returned to the reception to settle their dues. This time they encountered another gentleman in his late thirties with a borrowed moustache who obligatorily asked if they had enjoyed their stay to which a very affirmative reply was provided, both by Freida and James.

They took his leave and left with assurances that they would return again.

Walking back towards the car James had an afterthought after yesterday's discussion and sex with Freida. He thought that maybe, once sex was invented by evolution, with male and female forms of life appearing and with combinations of their genetic transmission occurring, it was possible that true death of the parent organism became possible. Prior to that with binary division there was no death. This time he kept the thought to himself. Perhaps it may be foolish. He needed time to dissect it.

On the way home James played *Slim Dusty*'s *A pub with no beer* and *Waltzing Matilda* which sent both their vocal chords to full volume all the way home. Later they reminisced the day, with James thanking her for planning a great weekend, "We should this more often."

"Of course we will," she replied.

"Not next weekend, I have to meet your parents. I am so looking forward to it. I want to meet the makers of you."

"Sure, but there are no other offspring to meet."

You don't have any brothers or sisters?"

"No."

"You know, I have a sister, Janet who knows everything"

"Women usually know everything, except quantum physics"

"Maybe you will allow me to teach you some."

"Another time another place and another planet

maybe."

"Touché. You mass of sexual energy'

"You are no less mister quantum"

By the time they got to her apartment it was early evening so they made plans to go to dinner on the Newcastle Wharf. They would take her car and she would drive. They would stroll along the ferry wharf and have a few drinks at the pubs before and then find a nice restaurant.

They found a pub which was sufficiently not crowded. Both of them got beers and sat at a table determined not to attract attention.

"I enjoyed our weekend," James started.

"It was nice."

"Hey can you get a peculiar smell?" James inquired.

"It must be my perfume."

"No."

"It must be my pheromones."

"Are you trying to tell me something?" James asked

"Maybe my body is."

"Touché."

"You know what pheromones are?"

"Yes but please revise it for me."

"Pheromones are infochemicals between the same specifics whereas allelochemicals convey information among different species. Maybe the kangaroos and wombats were trying to tell us something at the vineyards," Freida continued.

"But why the smell now?"

"Maybe there's an animal around trying to compete with me for your attention,"

James smiled and decided to pull his foot out of his mouth.

After they had consumed their beers, they found an elegant Italian restaurant to satiate their appetites. Both of them favoured Risotto. She chose the *Asparagus and Prosecco Risotto* and he preferred the *Saffron Risotto with Prawns and Sea Urchins* nursed down by a bottle of Pinot Grigio. The food was delicious and required their undivided attention for full gustatory appreciation. As a ground ritual they shared the tastes of their choices.

"I think your choice is creamier." Freida observed.

"Between Italian and French I prefer French cuisine," James added

"I don't think we have any authentic French restaurants here."

"This is true. The French use a lot of butter in their cooking and yet they do not put on weight."

"How come?"

"I don't know. Perhaps it is their genetics or maybe they have small frequent meals."

"Yes you never find any bulky French but you do find many bulky Italians."

"I had some really nice snails which they call escargot and frogs legs when I went to Paris."

"Now you are making me jealous."

"Sorry, stop, cut."

They walked hand in hand to the car. Freida drove back. After a coffee at her apartment they parted with the usual hugs and kisses ritual. James had busy morning next day at his rooms. It had been a very good weekend after a very long time. Next weekend was planned to meet her parents. He wondered what may be in store there.

13

On the following Saturday as arranged, visiting Freida parents was on the agenda. Freida had informed her parents they would arrive for lunch.

They left in James' car and followed the Pacific Highway south towards Sydney. As the wheels gained speed, James attempting hard to discourage his tongue roll asked her, "Do you like *Charlie Pride*?"

"*Charlie Pride*? I love him."

"I thought you loved me," he tried to hit a confirmatory note to allay his own thoughts.

"I love you much much much more," she reached out and kissed him.

"And guess what?" she added.

"What?"

"*Freedom is just another word for nothing left to lose*," reciting the words from the *Charlie Pride*'s song, *Me and Bobby McGee*.

"How true. Here's, *Me and Bobby McGee* just for you."

"Thank you."

Both of them accompanied the song at the top of their voices.

When the song subsided, "Charlie would be proud of us," she remarked.

"I don't think so. He would be jealous of you. Not me. You sing very well," James complimented her.

"And so do you," she echoed.

"Do you want to listen to *Is anybody goin' to San Antone*?"

"Or Phoenix Arizona," she hummed on.

The song followed and both of them belted to the capacity of their lungs again.

More Charlie Pride songs followed and with their duo voices contributing, they closed in on the red stone sides of the highway at Mount Colah soon.

They drove to her parents' house at Asquith near Hornsby. As they were driving down her street some school uniformed girls were laughing on their way to school up the road.

She pointed to them and, "I wore that uniform for six years at school."

"Why are they at school today?"

"They are the gutsy Saturday detention crowd," she explained.

"Do you ever wear that label?

"No, I was a very obedient girl at school. Always heeded the restrictions."

"Do you think school uniforms are a good idea?"

"For girls definitely. It removes the pressure of deciding what to wear every morning and the stress of competing for attention and meeting the expectations of your peers."

"For boys, I can say it enhances a sense of mob belonging and pride. I remember our mantra at interschool footy matches. Someone would start, 'Two, four, six, eight. Who do we appreciate?' And then we would all shout in chorus 'St. Pauls' again and again till our voices gave up."

"That's a boy thing."

"At St Pauls, usually, the 'I know it all' padres were teaching the 'I know more than you' boys. Me included. The parents of course were the eternal referees. I enjoyed my time at school. I read a lot of books from the school library."

"Do you like to read?" Freida inquired.

"Very much so."

"Who is your favourite author?"

"I have several favourite authors"

"One please."

"If you really really pushed me I would say Sommerset Maugham."

"Wasn't he homosexual?"

"We don't know. It does not matter to me."

Freida understood. So far so good she thought.

"What about you?"

"I like Jane Austen mostly but I also like George Eliot and Joseph Conrad."

"So you get to mention three. You allowed me only one."

"Okay tell me your others"

"I like Virginia Woolf and Fyodor Dostoyevsky and Charles Dickens."

"Who doesn't like Charles Dickens? Have you read '*Bleak House*?'"

"I read it in school. I remember liking it."

"Hey, drive slowly now. It's that house coming up on the left," she pointed.

They arrived outside the house, which had a high white cement rendered brick fence wall with a two way gate which was left open obviously in expectation of their arrival.

The peach blossom oleander bushes within seemed

to welcome them with their beautiful lance-shaped, waxy dark green leaves and their large whorled pink flowers providing a quasi-apricot fragrance to the vicinity.

When James had parked on the street outside the house, Freida jumped out of the car and raced in with the bottle of claret they had brought. She looked back and yelled out to James, "Follow me," which James did with some perceivable apprehensiveness.

Her mother came to the door and imparted Freida a hug.

"Any problems on the way?" she asked.

"No mum, all is well. This is James, short for doctor Regan,"

"Hello James, Freida has told me all about you."

"Freida, how could she know? I only met her on the way here," he rolled his tongue to answer and laughed. She echoed an obligatory laugh to reinforce his humour.

"She told me you are very good at your work in plastic surgery. I think I could use some of your services."

Her mother was slightly shorter than Freida with short clipped sandy brown hair but unlike Freida her nose appeared to have evolved to restrict the ambient smells rather than breathe. Nevertheless she had the elements of beauty which had been generously genetically imparted to Freida. She wore gold rimmed glasses and gold earrings that hung like stalactites almost from the concaves of her ears. James could not exactly decipher why his services would be needed at all, unless she had a body dysmorphic disorder. He sincerely hoped not. But then some women are crazy, self-obsessed, or vain. He remembered Ira Bunting. He would hate to have Ira Bunting as a mother in law. He must watch Freida's mother closely.

When they went in, her father was sitting on the sofa apparently deprived of any utility. His attempts at balding were achieving fruition except for some strands of white hair in the nuchal region that seemed determined to fight an eviction notice. His eye visors which were almost dropped were suddenly raised when he was disturbed by the black groodle that announced the arrivals.

The groodle attempted to seek James' upper torso for perhaps a kiss and James appeared unimpressed. He thought about the allelochemicals they had talked about recently.

"Leo, go away," Grace yelled at the groodle. The groodle awaited a manual interpretation of the order and was obliged by a light slap on the rear by Grace. The groodle understood this to mean that he was to rest at Frederick's feet and measured his length there.

"Fred this is James," Grace walked swiftly towards Fred who was still attempting to gain some consciousness. James followed her.

Fred got up and adjusted his hearing aids into his ear canals. He held out his hand to James and introduced himself, "Frederick George."

"I am very pleased to meet you sir," James said rolling his tongue again.

"Sit down my boy," Fred pointed to a sofa seat next to his.

"Thank you."

James acclimated to the sofa as instructed.

"How are you?" James asked.

"I'm grand," Fred replied.

Freida had also warned James that her father had an infinite capacity for remembering things that never happened. With this information at hand James was afraid to initiate a deeper conversation and spent the moments visually admiring the groodle. The groodle reciprocated. Fred himself appeared not to mind the ambience of the moment, perhaps also dictated by his deficient hearing.

Meanwhile Freida and Grace found their way to the kitchen and returned with some glasses and the bottle of claret, some cheeses and nuts. Grace poured the wine into the glasses and passed them around. When she had finished they raised their glasses and uttered "cheers" in unison before starting to sip the contents and expressing their individual delights and agreements on the wine.

"Tell me have you been watching the cricket, James?" Fred inquired. The wine appeared to have a provoking effect on Fred's vocal apparatus which was now set in motion.

"Sorry I am not a great fan of cricket. I like American football. That is my game and I root for the Falcons." He had researched that last night. Freida who was eyeing him closely responded with a smile. Freida knew that she had found her man. James did what he was told to do!

"Brutal game played by brutes. Cricket is such a

gentlemanly game," Fred responded.

"Yes but it takes five days to get a result and sometimes even that is not long enough in cricket," James argued.

"I agree you have to be patient but every moment can make you hold your breath."

James decided not to pursue the subject but continued to roll his tongue and nod as if in partial agreement.

"I know you are a doctor but what is your turf?" Fred inquired.

"I am a plastic surgeon," James answered.

"Good thing we don't have the fireplace on," Fred laughed.

Another dad joke, he thought and produced a prevaricated laugh.

"So what do you do now?" James asked him.

"I watch birds now."

"The feathered ones," Grace was quick to intervene for fear of misinterpretation.

"I worked for the Commonwealth Bank for fifty years. I started as a teller right after high school and finished as a bank manager. I retired about six years ago."

'No Fred it was seven years ago," Grace corrected, "I remember we had some flood claims that year at work."

At this point the groodle got up and walked towards James. James patted Leo on his head and inquired of the dog, "So how are you Leo?"

The dog appeared to appreciate his concern and attempted to lick his hand.

"Leo is very friendly. The kind of dog you would

want if you had no time to show intruders around. Leo does that very well," Grace added.

"We should be having lunch soon. I am famished," Freida got up from her seat.

They emptied themselves from the lounge room and assembled in the dining room which was adjacent to the kitchen, led by Freida.

Fred released his gluteal region into the chair at the head of the table and Grace dutifully occupied the foot end. Freida and James sat opposite each other.

Lunch was roast duck with peeking sauce and roasted carrots, beans, potatoes and peas with sesame seeds.

"This is good. I like the sauce particularly. It is sweet and spicy. Did you make it?" James asked Grace.

"Hell no. A Chinese friend of ours, Meng who lives down the road brought me some this morning. It is called hoisin sauce. It is made from soybeans, and spices. She makes it herself. Meng introduced us to Peking duck."

"Meng's daughter, Sue was with me in school," Freida informed James.

"How is Sue going mum, do you know?"

"She had her second son recently," Grace informed her.

"I like Chinese food particularly the sweet and sour pork," James confessed.

"I love the char siu barbecued pork. I remember when Meng used to invite me over she always made char siu."

"We have had Chinese cuisine in this country for as

long as I can remember. The Chinese restaurants create magnificent dishes all around the world. I had some great Chinese and Indian food in England. Indian food is also very good. We should go for Chinese soon in Newcastle, Freida," James said.

"Fred and I are not great disciples of Indian food. We find it too pungent for our tastes," Grace said.

The food conversation was beginning to gain dominance, Fred noted.

"Meng's husband is an accountant. I often get to pick his brain when we meet," Fred was feeling left out and offered his contribution for a shot at diversion. However his attempt was futile and Grace had her way.

"How long have you known James, Freida?" Grace asked.

"A very long time," Freida lied.

"But you never said a word to us."

"He also works at the Royal Hospital," Freida informed.

"So I don't have to guess where you met"

"My family comes from Ireland," Fred interrupted.

"Dad, James and I have been through all that."

"My ancestors are from Edinburgh in Scotland. I have some close relations in Dunedin in New Zealand. Fred and I visit them sometimes. They always take the mickey out of Fred with enthusiasm for being Irish. He does not seem to mind. Do you Fred?" Grace shouted toward Fred.

Fred leaned closer and provided a deepening of his nasolabial grooves to denote concurrence.

"I have never been to New Zealand. I would someday like to visit the birthplace of Lord Rutherford of Nelson. He has been my idol since childhood," James said.

"Who is he?" Grace wanted to know.

"He is a Nobel prize recipient for his work on radiation and nuclear physics," James informed.

This was getting a bit heavy going now both for Fred and Grace.

"Have you been to Ireland James?" Fred try to divert the conversation.

"Yes, when I worked in England a few years ago, I took a trip there."

"Grace and I visited several years ago too. We hired a car and drove around. The Ring of Kerry was magnificent. I can still remember the views. We also visited western Europe at that time. Grace loved Paris. I have fond memories. Freida was only a baby. She does not remember the trip," Fred went on.

"No Fred we did not hire a car and drive. We took the bus coach tour around," Grace corrected.

"Really. I always thought we drove."

"Dad, James and I are planning to go to Ireland sometime," Freida said.

"Good on you. I am sure you will see people there who knew our ancestors," Fred added.

"James has relations there too," Freida said.

After some more jejune talk to include the mundane concerns of everyday life, Fred excused himself to indulge in his afternoon siesta appointment, "I will see you next time, James. It was nice meeting you today. I will catch up on American football in the meantime if I can. Forgive me if I forget. My memory is not so good these days, so they tell me."

"You don't have to just for my sake," James replied.

Fred retired to his bedroom and was soon asleep as manifest by the emanating snoring.

"Just for the craic should we have some port?" Grace asked.

"Not for me, I have to drive," James said.

"Not for me too," Freida added.

The conversation next shifted to James and his parents. James informed Grace that his ear nose and throat father, Rodney was due to retire soon and become a vigneron. His mother, Elena who was an audiologist would accompany him to the vineyards. His sister Janet was a teacher and was still not romantically attached.

"Well if she is as attractive as you she should have no problem," Grace said.

"She is not short of risk takers. She claims she is not ready for a serious relationship yet," James replied.

"All marriages involve some risk. As long as the risk is not substantial. There is no virtual certainty except in Indian and Italian marriages," Grace humoured.

Precisely at this moment James was panged with the thought of Carmen and her baby. He was able to glide out without any facial betrayal.

"You are very wise. Is Freida as wise as you?" James asked.

"She has her glorious moments," Grace laughed.

"And very many of them," Freida added.

"I will make some tea," Grace volunteered.

"Not for me please," James replied.

Grace appeared confused.

"We have to be going, mum, James has some

patients to catch up with."

"Okay, take care, both of you and you Freida please try ringing me just to test if my phone works."

"Sure mum."

They got up to leave.

"Okay, bye, bye, bye, bye, bye" Grace continued.

On the way back the conversation was a concatenation of otiose hospital happenings. When that fuel ran out, "Next time it is your turn to meet my family," James said.

"I would very much like that and very soon I hope," Freida agreed.

It appeared ostensible to James that Freida had similar thoughts as him.

Back at Freida's apartment their immanent sexual appetites were aroused and the appropriate coitalbatic acts were requisitioned. Subsequent to showering together they decided to seek a fast meal at the local Macdonalds before parting for the night.

It was arranged to see James' parents at Warners Bay on the following Saturday for lunch.

14

It was Saturday and the meeting with James' parents was due. They picked a bottle of merlot and some roses and chocolates on the way.

His parents lived on a two acre property at Warners Bay with two horses and a dog.

The jacaranda trees in the ranch style fence yard in front had laid their lilac flower carpet to welcome them on their arrival and provided their unique faint aroma to the atmosphere. James mentioned to Freida that once, when he was gainfully employed at home in his younger days, it was his duty to rake the purple flowers. And how he did not look forward to that job every time! She told him that the jacaranda flowers at Sydney University heralded the impending arrival of the apocalyptic exams and time to stop partying!

Elena met them at the door. Elena was in her late fifties and appeared not to challenge the aging process. In profile the integument from her chin ran straight to the upper end of her sternum without any hesitation for a transverse interference by any form of wrinkling.

"Mum, this is Freida. She works as a research scientist at the hospital," James introduced Freida.

Elena was impressed by Freida's appearance and complimented her, "You look great Freida and your dress does you justice."

"Thank you," Freida responded. It seems her efforts at beautifying herself that morning were appreciated. She was wearing an orange polyester silk top and a blue maxi skirt.

"Please come in and sit down. Rodney has gone to the shops to pick up some food. He should be back soon."

Freida and James occupied the nearest three seater sofa. Elena took her place in one of the other single seaters.

"Make yourselves comfortable," Elena said.

"How have you been mum?" James inquired.

"Very well," Elena replied.

As prophesied by Elena, Rodney was back with some cheeses and wine. Rodney was pushing his early sixties and walked with a slight pendulous swing. He had a full head of hair which had been admonished recently by a comb. The hair colours combatted for hues of white. The hair at the nape turned back upwards for more sunlight perhaps. He had the familial chin dimple. He rolled his tongue and uttered, "Who is this beautiful girl you have with you James?" He eyed her closely. "Wait a minute. You are one that's raising the beauty index at the hospital and you really don't need a plastic surgeon do you? But considering it is James I shall let it pass. Congratulations James."

"Thank you Dr. Regan," Freida responded noting the tongue roll was possibly familial.

"Call me Rodney, Rod for short," he rolled his tongue again.

"Okay Rod."

"Where's Mercury?" James inquired.

"She said she could not make it today," Elena replied.

"She's always busy," Rodney added for completion.

"Who is Mercury? Freida inquired.

"That's James' name for Janet," Elena explained.

"Like Mercury, Janet is always going in the opposite direction," James added for explanation.

"I am going to open a bottle of Bordeaux Cabernet Sauvignon. This has a beautiful aroma of plums, blackberries and olive and not much tannin. I have some blue camembert to compliment it. Okay with you Freida."

"Sorry Rod, I am not a connoisseur in these matters," Freida replied.

James intervened, "You will lose points here if you say that. Best to say, 'I would really like to try that' and then pretend to look, smell the glass and taste and then think for a moment and utter 'that's a nice drop', even if you don't like it". But I can guarantee you dad's choices. You will be okay."

"I will go by what you say James. I trust you too, Rod."

"All agreed then," Rodney completed.

Rodney brought in some wine glasses and opened the bottle. He passed the first glass to Freida.

"Remember what James said, look for clarity and colour, smell the fruit, taste the sweet, salt or bitter. Is it thin like skim milk or full body like whole milk? The more alcohol the more the body and finally look for the finish, how long the taste lasts for. Does it last for a short or long while? That's all there is to it. The rest is prose."

"Thank you Rod. That was very informative for me."

"No problem."

They sipped the wine slowly.

"Tell me about yourself Freida. Are you from Newcastle?" Rodney asked.

"No, I am from Sydney. I graduated from Sydney University and eventually got a doctorate from there. Now I am doing research in comparative facial defects."

"That sounds interesting. Do you like animals?" Elena asked.

"Yes, particularly cats. They are so lordy."

"We have a basset hound here. Where's Nap gone? Nap we have a visitor," Elena attempted to raise her voice a bit in the diection of the kitchen.

"Nap? That's an interesting name. Does he sleep all the time?" Freida inquired.

"That too. But our Nap is short for Napoleon."

"I'll go find him," Elena disappeared.

Nap was found napping in the main bedroom. On being woken up from his daily schedule of sleeping, the dog followed Elena dutifully to find out what his next task was.

When he saw Freida and James he provided his obligatory bark and attempted to befriend Freida. Freida patted him gently establishing her 'friend' position with the dog.

"Okay Nap that's enough," Rodney intervened.

The dog knew that when Rodney spoke it meant 'settle down' and he chose to settle near Elena.

"You guys must be hungry. Let's eat," Elena made towards the kitchen.

In the dining room, Elena introduced her culinary attempts, "I have cooked some *veal scallopini with mushroom sauce*. I hope you like it."

"I love veal," Freida said.

"Mum did that on purpose. She knows I love her scallopini with mushroom sauce."

"The cabernet sauvignon will go nicely with veal. I will open another bottle," Rodney went off to find another bottle.

When he returned the glasses were re-equipped.

The meal was punctuated with the usual "beautiful", "lovely" and other such remarks with Elena accepting the compliments with the usual 'thank you'.

"We have cheesecake for dessert," Elena offered.

"Nice. That's great," Freida said.

The cheesecake looked lovely.

"Did you make it?" Freida inquired.

"Yes"

"Can't wait," James said.

After the meal, Freida helped to clear the table and load the dishwasher and set it in motion.

"You must see our horses later, dear. Do you like horses?" Elena inquired.

"Yes I do, but I was not allowed to ride. One of my cousins fell off her horse and had to have back surgery. She still tends to limp a little. Ironically he name is Eileen," Freida told them.

At the end of the meal satiety reigned and they retired to the lounge room with Rodney offering them all some tawny port.

Elena came in later with some Godiva Belgian chocolates and offered them to Freida first.

"I love chocolates" Freida ecstasised.

"The chocolate drink was first discovered by the Mayans and the Aztecs in Central America. They called it *shocoatl,* hence chocolate. The parent cacao plant has its pods growing straight from the trunk. This tree played a part in their spiritual lives. From those beginnings the Belgians and Italians I think now have the best chocolates in the world," Rodney informed.

There was a ring at the door and Elena got up to answer the door.

"Guess who is here?"

Janet came in, "Hi mum"

She entered into the lounge. She was dressed in a short sleeve yellow blouse and purple pants and wore her head in a bun.

"Sorry I am late. I have already had lunch."

"We have some left over if you feel hungry," Elena offered.

"No mum. I am fine."

"I can pack some for you to eat later if you wish."

"No mum my fridge is full. How are you dad?" Janet inquired.

"I am fine. It good to see you, darling," Rodney said.

"How are you? I want you to meet Freida," James interrupted.

"Hi, It's so nice to meet you," Janet responded.

"Nice to meet you too, Janet," Freida replied.

"So where did James find you Freida?" Janet inquired.

"I work at the hospital. I am a research scientist," Freida replied.

"So how are you Mercury?" James inquired of Janet.

"Fine, my dear moon," Janet responded.

"I can see you are all an astronomy family. But why moon?" Freida wanted to know.

"You can only see the one side of him. The other side is never in view," Janet explained.

Freida felt slightly worried but she did understand the complications of sibling relationships. Irrespective, she wished she had a younger sister. She would definitely have adored a younger sister. But a brother, that would not be bad either, she thought.

"Well, mum is mother earth and dad is Jupiter," Janet explained further.

"But where's you sun?" Freida questioned.

Rodney was impressed by the question. As if on cue just at this moment Nap who had vacated the lounge earlier reentered.

"There's our sun. While he naps we all move around him," Elena laughed.

"Good analogy mum" Janet complimented.

The conversation now sedimented toward the weather and the expected rain.

"We should be going soon," James said.

Elena saw an opportunity, "Freida before you go would you like me to pack some food for you?"

"No mum, Freida is on a diet. Like Nap she only eats one meal a day," James intervened.

"She can put it in the fridge and eat it tomorrow."

"No mum we are going out tomorrow," James continued.

"As you wish. You know that those restaurant

meals are not healthy."

"We'll manage. We need to be going soon, I have some patients to catch up with."

"Can she say hello to Mork and Dindy?" Elena asked.

"Okay, but don't take too long," James replied.

"Okay, come with me Freida," Elena led the way to the backyard acreage.

"The black stallion you see is Mork. Mork is a purebred Arabian. He is gelded. The little mare is Dindy, his daughter. Her mother was pure Egyptian Arabian. I have had them for a long time," Elena explained.

"They are beautiful horses. Do you ride them?" Freida fondly patted both of them.

"No, both Rodney and I have problems that come with growing up."

"Then what do you do with them?"

"Just love them. They have been with us for so long. We can't let them go."

"Fair enough. We better join James and Rod. James is in a hurry."

And they went inside again.

James was up and waiting, "Finished? Did Mork and Mindy say anything?"

"Yeah, they said James visits but never comes to say hello to us," Freida laughed.

"Ah well. Such is life. They still have things to learn," James closed, heading towards the door, followed by Freida and Elena.

"Bye Janet, see you sometime," Freida waved.

"Bye Freida," Janet responded.

"The meal was delicious. You are a fantastic cook," Frieda complimented Elena and rewarding her with a hug.

"Thank you for the wine and the wine information," Freida waved to Rodney.

"It was nice to meet you Freida. Obviously we will see more of you no doubt," Rodney replied.

On the way home in the car Freida commented, "I like your family"

"Yeah, dad has some arthritis and is forever cranky. Perhaps because of the pain. Mum as you may have noticed tries to off load her cooking on to anything that moves."

"I like that you are an astronomy family. I like astronomy. I want to take it up as a hobby soon."

"Good idea. All you have to do is look up at night first with the unaided eye, then with binoculars and then with a telescope. It's best to get to know the night sky first, identify a few anchor objects like planets or constellations that help you navigate the sky, and then go for a telescope. Generally, the best time for stargazing is when the moon is in a crescent or gibbous phase or when it's not present in the sky at all."

"Interesting."

"If a bright light in the sky sparkles, it's a star. If it doesn't and appears stationary, it's a planet. The path that the sun takes in the sky is called the ecliptic plane. Several of the planets, follow this same path. In other words, if you trace the ecliptic plane you can find most of the planets."

"You know a lot James."

"Yes, my dad kept us curious about it right from the time we were little."

"How did we get names like Mercury, Venus,

Jupiter and the like?" Freida asked.

"About twenty thousand years ago, there was nothing you could really do to control nature. It was very unpredictable. So, in order to establish some sort of control, humans attributed gods to nature. That way, they could have a sort of dialogue with nature and, thus, a measure of control. The oldest civilizations created that relationship with nature through god myths. Rituals were a way of establishing this dialogue with the gods. Once started this naming tradition continues, it persists even till today, even with our modern scientists. It's like in particle physics when Murray Gell-Mann called them quarks, because they were quirky particles that were not directly observable. Do you remember:

Three quarks for Muster Mark!
Sure he hasn't got much bark
And sure any he has it's all beside the mark from James Joyce's, *Finnegan's Wake*"

"Sorry, I have not read much James Joyce," Freida admitted.

"He has some nice works, *Ulysses, Dubliners, A Portrait of the Artist as a Young Man,*" James continued.

"I promise to read him."

"I have copies of *Dubliners* and *A Portrait of the Artist as a Young Man* in my room at mum and dads. We can pick them up when we next go there. But always make it much after lunch time. Or else food awaits the unwary."

"I understand. I will remind you," Freida said.

"Continuing on our initial topic, the ritual tradition persists only in the religions now."

"It's amazing how we have made such great strides

in astronomy," Freida added.

"Humans are curious creatures. We live just to want to know."

"The really brave Copernicus put us on track here," Freida added. She was also interested in the history of astronomy herself and its discoverers.

"Kepler, Galileo, and Newton then plodded on to get us here," he added.

"Don't forget Tycho Brahe. I love his name. It's like a boxer's name. And in the red corner all the way from Denmark we have Tycho Brahe with his precise and frequent observations of the planets and the stars."

"You are right there Freida. I love the way you put it."

"Did you know there is water on the moon?" Freida informed.

"Yes, water is found in the shadowed craters of the Moon and also on Mercury. Uranus and Neptune are made mostly of water. The water we have today was most likely delivered to Earth through impacts by small icy bodies perhaps tens of millions of comets, and even asteroids."

"Wow, I didn't know that."

"Did you know that Jupiter is the biggest of all the planets and Mercury is the smallest?"

"That I do know."

"Did you know that it rains sulfuric acid on Venus?"

"That might not allow *Gene Kelly* to sing in the rain to *Debbie Reynolds* on the romance planet. Ha ha"

"Io, one of Jupiter's moon is the most volcanically active in the solar system and is a terrible polluter, spewing sulphur and other material all over.

Ganymede is the largest moon in the solar system, and it's even bigger than the planet Mercury," James continued.

"Ganymede is another of Jupiter's moons along with Europa and Callisto right?" Freida asked.

"Yes and Callisto is the most bashed up guy in the solar system."

"Time to run rings around Saturn," Freida humoured.

"Yes those rings are name alphabetically in order of discovery. The largest gap in those rings is called the Cassini division."

"What about Uranus?"

"Uranus is the only planet that orbits on its side"

"Like lying on a boat and sailing down the Rhine like my mum wants to do," Freida said.

"Sort of. And Pluto is smaller than our Earth's Moon and also rotates on its side with Charon."

"We seem to have similar interests," Freida admitted to James.

"We are not done yet. We have not covered asteroids and comets. But just for the records, Halley's Comet completes a full orbit about every seventy-six years."

"*One, two, three o'clock, four o'clock rock*" Freida started.

"*Five, six, seven o'clock, eight o'clock rock*" James continued.

Then they both continued at the acme of their voices, "*Nine, ten, eleven o'clock, twelve o'clock rock We're gonna rock around the clock tonight……..*"

Almost panting for breath James started again, "*You shake my nerves and you rattle my brain*"

And together they continued,

"Too much love drives a man insane
You broke my will
But what a thrill
Goodness gracious, great balls of fire!
I laughed at love ....."

The singing continued till they got to Freida's apartment.

They decided they would go for a Chinese meal but till then they had work to do in the bedroom first.

15

Some weeks later they decided to go for a picnic to Barrington Tops close to the Upper Hunter. The drive was pleasant and this time *Harry Belafonte* took the music away in James' car with James and Freida' prompting and improvising.

They parked the car and found a nice spot to lay their own wares for personal consumption. Chilled beers were delivered straight from the bottle to the mouth, allowing no interaction with the surrounding rising temperature, to the mutual satisfaction of both the drinker and the bottle contents.

The black plumaged brush turkeys with their red heads and yellow throats observed the intruders from a safe distance, having their wings on alert for an emergency departure if the situation sanctioned.

"Isn't it a beautiful day? I'm glad we decided to venture here," Freida began.

"Indeed it is very relaxing but I am planning to stress you very soon," James responded.

"Don't be ridiculous I am not planning to take my clothes off here in front of all these people around. You better revise your plans."

"Hey settle down. That can wait for a moment."

"So what is really on your mind?"

"Do you really want to know? I want you to see no

evil, hear no evil and speak no evil after I finish."

She was trying to decipher what he meant by that. Was she about to be dropped? Surely he did not have to drive her all the way up here to convey that message. What is she to do just in case? She would not like to be in his car again or anywhere near him to get back home.

Suddenly he surprised her, "Freida, I have been thinking. Will you marry me?"

Freida had been hoping for this question eventually but not so soon. However she had her decision ready just in case. At this time it was a 'no brainer' for her.

Nevertheless, "What? I need to think about it. How long do I have? No, on second thoughts, yes provided we….," she pretended hesitating.

"Provided what?"

"Provided we have three children."

"Only three?"

"That'll do for a start."

"Now it's my turn to rethink, I need time to think about it. On second thoughts, yes."

"Well that's settled then."

"Shall we arrange for next month and a honey moon to Ireland?"

"And Paris on the way back?"

"Sure. That should be nice."

"James dear I'm so happy. Can I let mum know?"

"Definitely and let's fix an exact date by this evening."

"James you know I am not fussed on all that church crap? "

"Ditto."

"James I am so happy. "

"Would you like some more beer?"

"All the beer you can provide."

More bottles were consumed along with the cheese and tomato sandwiches that had been invited to accompany them on their trip, at the risk of consumption.

"We should celebrate tonight," Freida suggested.

"Sure, I will shout the evening."

After a while they packed and left after disposing the empty bottles in the nearby bin.

This time they needed no music accompaniment on the way back. They provided it themselves.

James went home to be ready for the evening. The times were beginning to change for both of them.

That evening at dinner they talked about the possible wedding roles list. James chose Damien White to be best man. Freida had seen him at the hospital and had no objections. Other roles were also allocated.

"I told mum about us. She was over the moon," Freida informed James.

"Freida, just for fun, you wouldn't consider a Hindu wedding, would you?" James humoured.

"But we are not hindus in a contractual marriage setting," Freida knew he was only pulling her leg.

"We don't have to be hindus. I am only talking about the *lagna* which is the ceremony."

"But darling, we would have to employ a hindu marriage celebrant who may refuse, we have to learn what to say without knowing exactly what it means, and get the invitees to wear Indian clothes etcetera. All this could take years. A Hindu marriage is a sacrament and fire is their only witness. I don't think neither you nor I could fall for that."

"You are right. I was only thinking of the pleasure of riding an elephant."

"I would love to wear a sari which I must admit may also take all your engineering skills to dismantle later in the bedroom. And knowing how patient you are! However I must admit it will be vibrant to watch but not for us, as participants."

"At least can we exchange garlands, do you think?"

"Yes that would be different. But I get to choose your flowers and you get to choose mine."

"We could start an australindian marriage ceremony tradition."

"But we still have rings."

"Of course. Is that a deal or no deal?"

"Deal."

The wedding was arranged for a Saturday at Meerans vineyard in Pokolbin. Although the weather was not very cooperative with threats of incidental precipitation, the marriage ceremony went boastfully beautifully with about seventy guests intending to make their presence felt. The vestiges of their australindian marriage ceremony intentions were visible in the decorative elements of the venue.

James wore a dark blue suit and a yellow polka dotted bow tie.

Freda looked magnificent in her white bridal satin gown which had a brilliant appearance and a thickness that provided volume. It was decorated with ribbons, organza and pleated lace details and she carried a bouquet of red and yellow roses. She wore three-inch heels visible at the bottom of the dress.

The male marriage celebrant, Cam was in his late forties as betrayed by his facial geodesics. He was attired in a dark brown suit and a red tie. He had a bespectacled formulaic face devoid of visible hair. His smile allowed an aeration of his upper gums. He was also imparted with a loud oratory voice requiring some elderly invitees to take their hearing aids out or to turn them off rather than risk a further hearing loss implicit in listening to his vacuous restricted attempts at humour.

At last to the couple's delight, "You may now kiss the bride was uttered," and the instruction was duly obeyed.

The nuptial ceremony subsided and the reception followed and the crowd was directed to marked tables. The hired master of ceremonies, Peter with his rudimentary attempts at humour took over. So far it had been a bad day for oratory humour. Fred, as the father of the bride was invited to "say a few words". Fred, with his hearing impediment, may not have heard the instructions as he had many more than a few words to say. Rodney next tested the patience of the microphone. The best man for the occasion was his cosurgeon, Damien White who set the crowd laughing by imitating James' mannerisms whilst delivering his speech with a rolled tongue. He also talked about how he first met James at a seminar when they were both residents with Damien being senior. When Damien had finished, by prearrangement a recorded Indian Bollywood song was played and Damien exhibited his *garba dancing* skills, setting the crowd now into full blown laughter.

And then the crowd were liberated to enjoy the food and alcohol which was served at the tables and the band betrayed its presence.

The guests enjoyed themselves, some more than others, aided by the alcohol.

Some exhibited their dancing prowess and others their dancing non prowess. James and Freida, of course were allowed to take the show away.

Due to work commitments, Ireland was dropped and James and Freida decided to honeymoon in Nelson in the South Island of New Zealand staying at the Rutherford Hotel named after Ernest Rutherford, the New Zealand nuclear physicist and winner of the Nobel Prize in Chemistry in1908. Freida worked this out as providing James a childhood dream for his honeymoon. James had always adored Lord Rutherford of Nelson.

Nelson remained tectonically quiescent during their stay. Sunshine attempted to purloin as much time as possible from the impending nights. Freida and James explored the surrounds as well as each other in the interim. They roamed the local beaches and national parks and tested the delights of the available seafood. They walked up to the top of Botanical Hill. The climb was steep requiring their deepest respiratory efforts at times. Along the way, they encountered some aspiring smocked artists with a cigarette in one hand and a paint brush in the other, attempting to set yesterday's wrongs to today's realism on the canvas, on their portable easels. The mahl sticks they brought along were mainly being used to deprive the watching wrens and cuckoos of a perch in the vicinity. Any attempted conversation with the artists invited magniloquent boasts of selling *sex* or *sivin* paintings to some unknown celebrities in the United States. When they reached the top, The Regans marvelled at the stunning views of Tasman Bay and the city. They noted that the Surveyors Needle structure pointing to the centre of New Zealand was huge.

"The view from here is beautiful," Freida remarked.

"Indeed it is. I am glad we walked up here. Going down should be easy"

"Yes but we must watch the potholes. Any misstep and the landing may not be compatible with life."

At the bottom they found a park bench to rest themselves and gain control of their respiratory debt.

When the situation was under control Freida started, "Mum said she thoroughly enjoyed our wedding ceremony and reception."

"A lot of our guests complimented us on the idea."

"It was your creative idea."

"It was your pragmatic solution."

In anticipation of expected questions from the guests concerning Hinduism dictated by the Hindu twist of their wedding, Freida had spent some time researching about its mythology and culture. She wished to discuss this further with James and note his views, "James, I want to talk to you a bit about Hinduism. I have done some reading. I think that what we call the Hindu tradition is really a fabric of civilization, weaving from various threads of religious life," she started.

"Yes, you are right. To me it seems the blending of Aryans from the north and Dravidians from the south, and the various tribal cultures resulted in a variety of religious practices. I think that this mixing of religious flows is better referred to as Hindu traditions rather just Hindu tradition," James continued.

"There are many sacred figures in Hinduism, each with many names and forms. Apparently this many-ness must be understood in relation to a radical one-ness, through the concept of Brahman which is one reality. So Brahman can be perceived in and through an infinite number of names and forms. Formulations and reformulations of these myths have continued through the centuries," Freida went on.

"Interesting isn't it? It is a concept that one has to accept. Like a rose is a rose is a rose, no matter what you call it. The earliest literary sources of the Hindu tradition are the *vedas*, literally knowledge, a body of ancient hymns and chants. The *Upanishads* consider the end of vedas and are their wisdom literature and take the form of dialogues between teachers and students, reflecting about the origin, basis, and support of the universe. Similar to the dialogue convention of instruction employed by Plato."

"Eventually things actually exist in the human mind in two ways, what exists in our understanding and what exists in reality," Freida summarized.

"Well put Freida. god exists in our understanding but not in reality."

"That's why we have different myths in different

religions."

"So we have rel-igion for understanding and we have real-igion for reality"

"Well put James. The mistakes the so called god made are being fixed by our scientists, doctors and lawyers today."

"Clerics, as you said learn only how to make better excuses for god and in doing so have to invent their own lies," James furnished.

Freida thought life could be interesting with James. James thought life could be interesting with Freida. Like minded they both were. Both looked forward to pursuing such issues further.

In the knowledge of Christianity common ground existed between them. James started, "In Christianity I have often wondered why the early church leaders were so dumb as to include four gospels, rather than just picking one?" James asked.

"Yes one would be good rather than create a schemozzle which finally reads as bullshit to me," Freida replied.

"The gospel passages are offered as a framework for a continuous portrait of Jesus' life from birth to death and resurrection. However this impression is somewhat misleading and really created by the early church fathers. If you have the time to read each of these gospels, much dissimilarity is easily apparent. The church is lucky the common man is unable or unwilling or does not have the time to read it for himself and think. And to aid his confusion further, they add latin, a dead language. And then the poor man has absolutely no leg to stand on."

"I have read the gospels. I did that some time ago when I was having problems with my beliefs. My friend Radia and I, did read and discuss them. You know Radia. She was at the wedding with her husband. Both her husband and she are vets. Radia is Polish and used to be a great catholic until she started to think. Both of us went through this together. Differences and even contradictions become so apparent when you actually read the gospels," Freida offered.

"Yes. Such differences actually question the historical veracity of the content of the gospels. Compare the genealogies of Jesus in the gospels of Matthew and Luke. Not only do the lists disagree, but Matthew is emphasizing Jesus' birth as following a pattern in which God intervenes dramatically in history on a very regularized basis, while Luke is emphasizing that Jesus' lineage goes back to Adam, son of God," James explained.

"Over the centuries, most Christians have tended to ignore the distinctive contradictions, and instead have scripturalized on these variations to address different or changing circumstances, to generate a theological creativity, or more really to construct polemics against other Christians or outsiders," Freida observed

"Exactly," agreed James.

"You find this in other Abrahamic religions too but Catholicism is the worst offender."

"Christian texts conflate selected elements into one single narrative, picture, or scene. I think it was *Tatian* in the second century who wove all four gospels into one single narrative, in the process eliminating doublets and fixing discrepancies.

Similar work had been in progress even before then," James went on.

"The New Testament reads all events as belonging to God's plan of salvation. This point is especially stressed through showing that events are the fulfilment of a prophecy, or through prophetic announcement. In addition, Christians used other modes of interpretation that were common in the ancient Mediterranean world, including allegory and elaboration. Many Christians emphasized a spiritual interpretation of scripture, while yet taking seriously the literal meaning and engaging constructively with contradictions and historical difficulties. My friend, Radia is an expert at identifying this. She showed me how this is done. We should get together with her," Freida continued.

"That would be good. Getting back, we should be thankful that Northern Europe underwent through all those series of social and intellectual changes during the period of colonial expansion and we should be eternally grateful to those individuals who pushed them. Thank heavens there was an increasing sense on the part of many intellectuals at that time that the key to truth lay in science and not in faith or tradition. These changes would have been kept under wraps by the infallible papa if he had his way. As a result biblical theology and interpretation in the West was profoundly affected by the Renaissance, the Reformations, the Scientific Revolution and the Enlightenment."

"Yes, the rise of scientific investigation brought to the fore a paradigm shift of how human beings can know about the world," Freida added.

"History writing was also impacted by science's high valuation of objective evidence as the basis for claims to knowledge and truth. Prior to this shift, history had been used primarily for edification, for example providing moral or political exemplars to imitate or to avoid and to offer cautionary reviews of past events to guide future action. I could continue talking on this forever," James added.

"Me too."

"I love such conversation."

"Me too."

James was happy. He had found a soul mate and Freida was happy too. She had found her sole mate.

James leaned closer and pecked her on her cheek, "I think we will have a good time together."

"If marriages were made in heaven, we would not have been allowed this conversation would we?" Freida commented.

"So where are marriages made then? I am at a loss to know."

"Right here on our planet Earth, in the bedrooms where the Jewish, Christian, and Muslim gods hang about and watch all the action," Freida continued.

'Have you read *Portnoy's Complaint* by *Philip Roth*?"

"No what's it about?

"It's about a young Jewish boy's obsession with masturbation, written with a great twist of comedy. It has to be read to be appreciated fully. It caused an outrage on publication."

"In that case it is a compulsory read for me. *Portnoy's Complaint* by *Philip Roth*."

"I think we did enough contemplated constructive thinking today."

"Indeed," Freida replied.

"Have you ever wondered with all the snow at Christmas, do shepherds really herd cattle in winter when there is no grass, for angels to appear to them and announce the birth of a saviour? Someone got that bitterly wrong apart from dates and not apples in the Garden of Eden in Mesopotamia," James remarked.

"I think we should find some ice cream," Freida suggested.

"Do they make date ice cream?"

"Let's find out."

They vacated the bench and sought their way into town in quest of date ice cream. Date ice cream? In New Zealand? In Nelson?

16

A month after their return back from Nelson, Freida realised that she was pregnant and decided to stop work. James secured her an obstetric appointment with Dr. Winston Woolard who had his consulting rooms at Hamilton. Dr. Winston was a middle aged man with a full head of black hair that was the envy of some of his clients' husbands. However his face bore the scars of many a sleepless nights, hopefully and dutifully spent in the obstetrics wards only.

Freida's pregnancy progressed in compliance with all the expectations of Dr. Woolard. A week prior to her delivery date, Grace came up from Asquith to stay and James continued to work. He had advised Freida what she should do in case he was not around at her due time. On the Wednesday morning when her contractions continued to last about one minute and occur every five to ten minutes apart, Freida knew her time was nigh. James was at work. She rang James and informed him of the baby's intentions and her impending moves. James told her that he would catch up with her at the hospital. A taxi was sanctioned which took Freida and Grace to the Mater Hospital at Waratah with her prepacked essentials.

A three and a half kilogram baby girl arrived in the afternoon with not much help from Dr Woolard who was present. He would have preferred to have been seen as being more useful. However his face did provoke the baby to cry and take its first breaths. In that sense he may be considered useful. The baby had blue eyes. When Freida held her the baby winked at her as if implying 'we're in this together'. Freida was a mother now. Her joy was great as witnessed by the look on her face. James was invited into the labour ward and allowed to hold the baby.

"She's beautiful," James enthused looking around for concurrence.

The midwife and Dr. Woolard nodded with smiles.

He kissed Freida,"Thank you my love."

"No problem. Plenty more from where that came," Freida chuckled. It was obvious that she was still in some pain.

James looked toward where Dr. Woolard was standing, "Hey Winston thanks for your help today but do you provide any bulk discounts?" James joked.

"Yes definitely. Upto a maximum of ten. But for deliveries during office hours only. For afterhours deliveries there is a surcharge for every hour after midnight," Dr. Woolard responded with a laugh.

The baby was carried outside the labour ward by James and allowed to delight Grace, Rodney and Elena who were waiting outside. Even Janet who usually could not be relied upon to be available within the hours of requirement was there.

Fred had been summoned to be in Newcastle from Sydney later in the day.

Freida and the baby were discharged from the hospital after two days with all the requisite instructions, from breast feeding to abdominal exercises and the follow-up visits.

At home Grace instructed Freida in baby and mother care with what she had learnt from her own mother, Alicia with appropriate *mutatis mutandis* applications. When the occasion provided, Elena took her turn educating Freida often with instructions that appeared to be in contradiction to those from Grace.

Regardless of these various unwelcome enforcements, the baby's homeostasis prevailed and she was always a happy and smiling baby. The parents had decided to name her Fiona.

Her every milestone was carefully followed by Freida to comply with Jean Piaget's stages. Freida had a camera ready to document her findings in case evidence was demanded. Fiona usually complied and was very infrequently argumentative. Freida took great pride in exhibiting the effects of her breast feeding on her produce to inquisitive passers-by, when she strolled down the streets with Fiona in the pram.

James' time was mainly harnessed by work commitments as his practice was still expanding. However when time and patience allowed he was happy to contribute.
Fiona continued to climb the ladder of development to both parents' extreme satisfaction and delight.

Soon little Fiona's perpetual curiosity demanded

more and more attention from Freida, which left Freida totally exhausted by the end of the day. James' nocturnal approaches were curtailed by Freida with the empress Joséphine Bonaparte's well known, "*J'ai mal à la tête*" technique. James understood.

Fiona's curiosity was unsurmountable. Everything interested her, from insects to rocks.

Both Freida and James encouraged her passion for knowledge. James remembered his own childhood when his father had a whiteboard installed at home to deliver answers to his own questions.

Fiona was more than ready for school at four years of age. However the state regulations interfered with an earlier entry. And besides, the schools and teachers likewise were not equipped to educate gifted children who were only considered a menace to an otherwise harmonious classroom.

Nevertheless Fiona did find school interesting and the teachers loved her.

A year later Faye arrived. Again, under Dr. Woolard's supervision she went through the same impositions that Fiona had been subjected to earlier. However Faye demanded more sleep time which pleased Freida but not Fiona. In her awake hours, Faye was aided by a doting elder sister who helped her in her grommet stages to ride some of the early waves. The sisters grew very close and always protective of each other in any adversity, either parent induced or otherwise.

In time, both James and Freida noticed that Faye

liked to be left alone and often had a pensive look. She learnt to read early and her questions usually had a 'what if' ring'?

"Dad, what if the earth was square rather than round?"

"Square and round is what you can draw on a piece of paper. What you mean is if the earth was a cube rather than a sphere, right?"

This set Faye thinking till James showed her a box and a football and the penny dropped.

"Well if the earth was a cube then when you come to the edge of one side, you would have to step to the other side before you continue walking. Like when you keep walking on flat ground until you come to a mound and you step above it to get to the other side."

"Oh yeah I know now."

More questions followed and neither Freida nor James ever felt perturbed.

"What if birds could talk just like us mummy?"

"Provided they spoke the same language as us we could understand them. Just like people. We do not understand people who speak a different language to us."

At four years of age Faye was also ready for school and wanted to accompany Fiona.

James' attempts were again rewarded by another pregnancy. This child however demanded separate terms of settlement and requested a caesarean birth. Freida endured her predicament with little complaint.

The elder sisters were joyed with the new addition and showered her with their unwelcome attention. Fatima as the new baby, demanded more attention from Freida. But now Freda's veterancy in baby management was in full control and soon Fatima realised that she was losing the power struggle and withdrew some of her time consuming demands.

Both elder sisters looked forward to playing with Fatima when they returned home from school.

Soon the local high schools for the elder sisters gave way to Sydney University one by one and Fiona graduated in physiotherapy and Faye finished speech therapy about five years after Fiona.

Both Fiona and Faye secured job appointments at Royal Newcastle Hospital in their respective departments.

The girls including Freida were very fond of Rodney and Elena and loved visiting them in their new habitat in the vineyards. Every so often they would go there on the weekends and the grandparents looked forward to their visits.

Today was a particularly warm day. On their arrival there, the air smelled anaerobic or close to rotten eggy when they encountered it, at the vineyard.
The three bedroom cottage located on the premises was a short drive from its frontage to the road, of the eight acre vineyard.

Rodney had now gained control of the vineyard and was a full winemaker or vintner. He often reminisced how the initial three years had been difficult year round work for him with his arthritis aided by pain killers. He had sometimes wondered if it had ever been a good idea. But then it kept him busy, physically and mentally. It was a challenge he loved. Dealing only with the council regulations for starting and running a vineyard would demand a few chapters if he ever wrote a book on the subject.

Although he had employed labour, the harvest involved long days and the so called 'dormant period' required other supporting activities in the vineyard including attending to machinery, some of which was obsessed with spending time in the company of other damaged machinery in the repair shops. He remembered the rare paediatric patient he had encountered who would refuse to go home because they had found a friend in hospital. It seemed to him at times that his grape harvester particularly, had had access to *Joseph Heller*'s *Catch-22* as it preferred to spend time at the repair shop rather than face the heat in the vineyard at Pokolbin. He was reminded of how *Captain Yossarian* and the others in the novel preferred spending time in hospital to flying the bombing missions.

The hired men on the vineyard often provided their own temperaments to complicate a bad day. Often their responses provided him an unplanned chance at inflicting morbidity but Rodney knew better.

He remembered the soil preparation and the tiring removal of any previous cultivation remainings and weeds, many weeks before the vines planting to which he contributed to the best of his disability. It also took a large amount of money and a lot of determination and work ethic that he was glad he possessed.

"How is school going Fatima?" Rodney inquired.

"Good. We are studying *Shakespeare* currently."

"Incidentally I have been to Stratford-upon-Avon, where Shakespeare was born and also died."

"How nice," Faye was impressed.

"Although Shakespeare worked in London at the Globe theatre, his wife, Anne Hathaway and his children lived in Stratford-upon-Avon. I went to see King Edward's School where he was educated. Which of his tragedies are you studying?"

"*King Lear*. I find it interesting. As you know it is a double plot in the stories of Lear and his daughters and Gloucester and his sons."

"Two fathers fall victim to the shenanigans of their children," James laughed.

"Man smart, children smarter," Freida laughed.

"No dear, *Belafonte* says, *Man smart, woman smarter*," James continued.

"It is like prodigal fathers reuniting with their own children sort of story," Fatima added

"I liked Cordelia and her stand. It is sad that she had to die at the end. Both men learn to see better the hard way, after trusting the wrong children," Grandma Elena remembered.

"All his tragedies repeatedly address tensions between the will and desires of the individual and the constraints emanating from his or her society," Rodney retraced back.

"The plays are consistently interested in the relationship between public and private life and in the emotional fissures within dysfunctional families," Grandma Elena added.

"In Shakespearean plays the different kinds of power is under negotiation. Political power, erotic power, the power of language and the imagination, and the power of theatre itself," Freida contributed.

"That's very well put Freida," Elena complimented Freida.

"To me, Shakespeare's protagonists articulate *in extremis*," James added.

"Yes James. That way the suffering of the tragic protagonist is rendered significant by the special insight or vision it allows him or her to achieve," Elena explained.

"Yeah mum, I see your point," James agreed.

"Mr Brown, our English teacher says we should admire the pity and fear it evokes and the catharsis or purgation it is meant to produce," Fatima said.

"I suppose so." James agreed.

"What about you? What do you think Fiona?" Elena asked.

Fiona thought for a while before replying, "Whatever".

"Shakespeare does have that effect on some people," Elena smiled.

"Is there any cause in nature that makes these hard hearts?" Fiona laughed.

"You must be patient," Faye finally contributed. Everyone looked at Faye. She had understood it much better. All she was saying is that humanity is trapped in a black, meaningless farce that must simply be endured patiently. Absurdity as Albert Camus deciphered is a better description, Rodney thought.

"It's time for lunch." Elena announced.

"You sit where you are Elena. The girls and I will

find something," Freida announced.

"I have some fried chicken in the fridge Freida. We just have to heat it up. Rodney will have a four'n twenty pie. You will find them in the freezer," Elena informed.

"I will have a pie too," Fatima said.

"Me too," Faye echoed

"Any more orders? What about you dad?" Fiona asked.

"I will have the chicken and any chips if we have."

"There is a pack of chips in the freezer on the left side Freida," Elena said.

"James would you like a drop of our recent Regan chardonnay?" Rodney inquired.

"Of course, anytime," James replied.

"You know James, it costs me less than two dollars to make a bottle of chardonnay."

"Really," a voice from the kitchen asked, possibly Freida.

Rodney vacated his seat with some manifest painful difficulty to fetch the wine from the cellar, singing to himself,

"Sing a song of sixpence
A pocket full of rye
Four and twenty blackbirds
Baked in a pie"

James and Elena and possibly the others were aware that Rodney did not appreciate being pitied for his mobility disability.

Faye appeared with some nut mixes, soy crisps and potato chips and placed them on the table in the middle closer to grandma and sat next to her.

"It's so quiet here grandma."

"Yes we did notice that very much initially when we moved. Rodney and I could actually hear each other. In recent years, the world has become more noisy through our human activities, traffic and industry noise, but also noise through our recreational activities."

"Traffic noise is usually low in frequency, and even birds in cities appear to sing with higher frequencies to prevent being masked. So we have soprano birds in the city and you must have tenor birds here."

"Yes, I ran into a *Luciano Pavarotti* yesterday," grandma chided.

Rodney came in with the bottles and glasses and placed them on the table defying temptations from gravity all the way. James did the pouring. The self-appointed chefs returned declaring lunch would be ready soon.

The Reagan chardonnay claimed some victory with James. It was a full-bodied, dry wine exhibiting a combination of berry fruit and oak notes, softer acidity, and a buttery texture.

After a couple of drinks the lunch venue was shifted to the lounge with each one bringing their plates in, except Rodney and Elena who were provided a waitress service. Just at this moment Nap stumbled in perhaps persuaded by his olfaction and settled near Rodney. In the course of ageing, Nap had allowed his abdominal anatomy to shift closer to the ground. Fatima and Faye imparted a part of their pie to Nap as a treaty for his continuing friendship.

"Rodney and I were invited to go sailing by Ernest Sab next weekend," Elena informed.

"What's Sabby doing these days?" James asked.

"After his wife died he went off the air for a while but luckily he has now recovered. He has a cabin cruiser and spends all his time repairing the monster. And when he is not doing that he sails," Rodney explained.

"Do you see him often?" James asked

"He does keep in touch. He is a good friend," Rodney finished.

"How is Mercury?" James asked.

"She comes sometimes with her boyfriend, Michael who is in the police force. He is a very nice polite gentleman," Elena said.

After a while it was time to go home.

"We should have a seafood barbeque next time. I will see if Janet and Michael can come," Elena said.

"That would be nice," Freida replied.

On the drive home an unnatural silence prevailed with everyone lost in their own thoughts. Freida was planning dinner. She had some barramundi which she could beer batter along with potato chips for tonight. James was thinking how much effort his father had put in the Regan chardonnay. It was not a bad drop, he thought. Fiona was thinking of Rodney's arthritis and if she could help him in anyway. Faye was thinking of Luciano Pavarotti singing to Grandma Elena. Fatima was having new thoughts on Shakespeare that she could impress Mr Brown with.

It had been a good day.

17

An opportunity arose for James to visit the Marshall Islands on a mission trip for two weeks. He wanted to discuss the matter with Freida alone but Fatima was also around when he got home.

"Would you like to come with me to the Marshall Islands Freida? I have an opportunity to do some charity work there for two weeks."

"Where is the Marshall Islands? I have never heard of them," Freida queried.

James had researched the matter,"They are a collection of five volcanic islands and twenty-nine coral atolls in the central Pacific Ocean, between Hawaii and the Philippines. They are named after Captain John Marshall who sailed through there with convicts bound for New South Wales."

"That sounds interesting. Are wives allowed?"

"I'm sure you can come if we pay your fare."

"Are the youngest child allowed? " Fatima asked expecting a negative reply.

James looked at Freida who looked the other way, implying, 'that's your decision James'.

James understood, "Provided you behave yourself and school allows."

"I promise to behave," Fatima agreed.

"Okay, you are in," James replied.

Fatima could not control her joy and immediately provided a jig to substantiate.

"The Marshall Islands were used by the United States to test their nuclear weapons in the forties and fifties. As a result of the radiation fallout the country has been left with a lot of birth defects that could employ my surgical skill. It could also provide beneficial experience for me."

"I'm very proud of you James," Freida said.

"Well, I am sure we will see a lot of cleft lip and palates, digit abnormalities, club foot and cranial defects. I could be very busy. Fatima and you can explore around on your own and see how the other side of the world lives."

"Do they speak English?" Freida wanted to know.

"No. They speak the Marshallese language also known as Ebon. It is not related to English. It is one of the Malayo-Polynesian languages."

"How will we understand them?" Freida queried.

"We will find a way. It will be an adventure," James replied.

"What? You Tarzan me Jane sort of?" Freida laughed.

"Will we be okay with the radiation? Is there any danger?" Fatima was anxious to know.

"That is a good question. I think we should be okay," James assured her although he was not sure himself.

"We can stop for a few days at Kauai on the way back to unwind. We can rent a car and drive around," he continued.

"Okay count me in," Freida agreed.

Fatima knew she was also included and favoured James with a smile.

Later James found out that between 1946 and 1958, the United States had used the Marshall Islands as an atom bomb testing ground. During that time, about 67 atomic bombs were dropped in the islands, on and around the atolls of Bikini, Enewetak, Rongelap and Utrik, while the Marshallese could only look on haplessly at this American self-acquired prerogative. Apparently Bikini and Enewetak atolls were still radioactive.

On being informed about the impending trip the elder girls were not particularly concerned, particularly because of their own work commitments. The necessary formalities were adhered to and the day finally arrived and they left from Sydney to arrive in Hawaii later in the evening. They spent the night in Hawaii and boarded the flight to Majuro the next day.

The plane had to make a stopover at Johnston atoll to refuel. The atoll was used as a base by the US and no passengers were allowed to get off the plane. Photography, even from the plane was also strictly prohibited.

On arrival at the Marshall Islands International Airport, known as Amata Kabua International Airport, three other passengers also alighted. The airstrip was basic and smelled heavily of diesel. They were garlanded at the airport by the local female beauties, some of whom left nothing to be not desired. This tradition apparently is bestowed on every visitor although it did make Fatima feel especially important as she aligned her head to ease the formality for the local girls. Something for her to report back at school. It would definitely make both Angela and Jean jealous. The airport was a mere tin shed, with a bench for travellers to sit the imposed no waiting and a table for the two officials who pretended to check the passports, converse with each other in ebon and stamp them. The Reagans were escorted by a Majuro Hospital car to their Marshall Island Resort hotel which was about 11 kilometres away.

Having unpacked and settled in their room they decided later in the evening to walk to the hospital and acclimatise themselves to the environs.

The denizens imparted them a nonchalantly despicable look as James, Freida and Fatima walked around as if these visitors were responsible for their current abjectivity.

"Dad why do they look at us like that?" Fatima wanted to know.

"That is called transference according to Sigmund Freud. A transfer of felt emotions, from their previous and actual target to a person currently present. The Marshallese feel the United States has betrayed their trust and failed to provide just compensation for the upheaval caused by the U.S. nuclear testing. Over the years the Marshallese have become dependent on U.S. aid and financing.

Freida and Fatima now understood the imbued antiamerican feeling now being imparted upon them. They fully understood the Marshallese feelings now.

Next morning after breakfast James walked to the

hospital and was met by the local medical superintendent who introduced himself as Dr Munisao Morean, who escorted James to the outpatients department where a multitude of semi clad patients awaited his arrival. Apparently some were waiting from the night before, as Dr Morean informed him. Notice was provided several weeks before to all the locals in the surrounding islands of a visiting plastic surgeon. It was obvious to James that this trip was going to be busy. The patients were instructed to come in fasting in case they needed imminent surgery.

Interpretation was provided by a local nurse equipped with the most basic reductionist English language knowledge. James was guided mainly by his inspection skills but he needed to take a history just for the records.

He saw a lot of raised thickened scars called keloids which are more common in dark skinned people. He knew that this is a difficult condition to treat. Surgery is sometimes performed. These cases were scheduled for surgery on the same day's afternoon list to be done under local anaesthesia.

The other operative cases were scheduled for the following days as appropriate.

The anaesthetist, Ivan Rosenburg was an American doctor with black wavy hair and an easily identifiable aquiline nose, who was spending a year in the Marshall Islands. He had a sense of humour when understood.

"So what brings you here Dr. Regan?" he asked.

"Just a break from routine work, I guess."

"Same class no glass."

James pretended he understood and provided a professional smile.

"What about you?" James inquired.

"Come to think about it, I really don't know. I'll tell you first if I ever find out."

Smug and cocky for sure. James will endure him for two weeks.

One evening, in the restaurant on the ground floor of the Majuro Hotel, Fatima appeared excited and burst out, "Dad I have been thinking and I have decided to become a doctor."

"That's great Fatima. What made you decide that?" Freida inquired.

"I saw all the people around here and felt that the world could really do with more doctors."

"Indeed, but to be a doctor you need to study and work very hard. I am sure you could do that if you really decided to be a doctor," James encouraged.

"You can easily do that Fatima," Freida helped.

"Deal," Fatima replied

"Radiation seems to cause a lot of thyroid disease here it seems," Freida said.

"They are the ones we see with large neck swellings isn't it?" Fatima asked.

"Yes," James replied.

"How does radiation act?" Fatima wanted to know.

"Radiation is an electromagnetic wave. You know what that means. You also know that the energy packed in a wave of electromagnetic radiation is directly proportional to its frequency. The higher the frequency is, the higher the energy. There are alpha, beta and gamma radiation waves. The most energetic are gamma rays. Of the ninety-two chemical elements, there are at least twenty eight elements that are radioactive that occur naturally on Earth. They have existed long before the solar system was formed," James divulged.

"The energy wave alters the replication of the cells and the effects can be transmitted to the offspring," Freida helped.

"Just remember PURT for Polonium, Uranium, Radium and Thorium which are the most common radioactive elements," James finished.

Fatima attempted to digest all the provided information.

The days passed uneventfully with the mornings devoted to outpatient sessions and the afternoons to operative schedules and no stressful or significant complications were encountered by James.

Dr. Morean organised a farewell meal for the Reagans, the evening before the day of their planned departure. The relevant clinical staff and the irrelevant bureaucrats were also invited. Dr. Rosenburg was also present. After the meal Dr. Morean thanked James for his services in his sententious speech. Dr. Morean attempted to practise his own oratory capacity further by also thanking the senior bureaucrats present. It was obvious that this speech had been delivered many times before with other visiting doctors.

Attempting departure from the island was an adventure in itself as the Reagans learnt. One had to present oneself at the airport when a stopover flight to Honolulu was expected and departure was only allowed if there were sufficient seats available on the plane. If there were not enough seats, one stayed on in Majuro till the next stopover flight was expected and then one tried one's luck again. But it was not only real luck that counted. Other forces, including the temperaments of the airport staff and the influential hierarchy of the traveller etcetera also mattered. Freida and Fatima gained an expertise in perpetually smiling at the probable airport staff and eventually seats were secured after two days of unfruitful attempts.

At Honolulu they took a half hour flight to Lihue Airport on the Island of Kauai and hired a car. James negotiated the right hand driving to Kauai Beach Resort where they had booked for five nights. Along the way, Freida provided the "*Aloha*" to the passing drivers who verbalised loudly their 'idiot on the road' chant. However James was very soon conditioned to the right hand driving.

"Kauai has the most beautiful beaches I have seen," Freida expressed her enchantments regularly.

Next day they started early as advised by the friendly hotel staff and James negotiated the very, very curved roads slowly to the Waimca Canyon Lookout with the greatest apprehension. The trailing traffic behind honked. He attempted to maintain the 'I also pay my taxes attitude' as much as possible. And they reciprocated with the 'not in this country attitude', as they had encountered many such, particularly British tourists before. Freida as usual provided the '*aloha*' spirit. He tried to go faster and the oncoming traffic honked. He resolved the dilemma in favour of safety by going slow.

The canyon views were spectacular. Freida suggested that they explore the waterfalls on foot which retrospectively was a bright idea. The walk took about an hour.

"The Waipo'o Falls are just magnificent," both Fatima and Freida maintained.

On the way back to the hotel they reminisced the day pleasantly. The local radio played music reminiscent from James' and Freida's school days. They joined in when *Petula Clark* contributed '*Never on a Sunday*'. Even Fatima who had been introduced to the song as a baby by Freida remembered the vestiges. James' driving had improved significantly as calculated from the verbal insults from fellow drivers which had declined to negligible levels and he was finally able to participate in the in-car conversation.

Soon Fatima's inquiry monitor prompted," Why do things, say some stories, some fashions, and some music become more popular than another?"

"Working that out, is the dream of everyone who has something to sell, a cause they believe in, or a message they want to spread," James said.

"Interesting question Fatima. Almost anything from products, political ideas, social movements, behaviours, fashion styles, diets or exercise trends, and even language can spread," Freida added.

"But why some and not others?" Fatima continued.

"Well, obviously most things that win out are just plain better than the ones that don't. We usually prefer products that are easier to use, drugs that are more effective and even scientific theories that are true rather than false," James explained.

"What effect does advertising have?" Fatima inquired.

"A lot. Advertising uses psychological and sociological mechanisms that make products, ideas, and behaviours catch on. How easy something is to try has a big impact on whether it catches on or not. That is why doctors get provided with free samples to try," James laughed.

"Our natural tendencies, drives, and motivations make us more likely to share some things rather than others," Freida contributed.

"Somehow some aspects of individual psychology make exactly the same drug less effective, when you get it at a discount price. Aspirin at fifty cents is less effective than the same aspirin for a dollar to some people," James added.

"Subtle cues in the environment can influence what we think about and how we behave. Remember how they play Christmas music in alcohol shops. Christmas and celebration and alcohol are associated in the human mind," Freida added.

"I guess there is also peer pressure to imitate and conform in individuals," Fatima added.

"Remembering is another factor. The more likely you remember a message, the more likely it is that you will tell it to someone else. Messages that are simple, unexpected, concrete, and credible are more likely to stick. Also repeatedly seeing and hearing the same message will make it stick. Who does not remember the Coca-Cola and Cadbury song messages on television with familiar tunes?

"Analogies also help make things simple, and memorable," Freida continued.

"Yes, analogies express new and complex ideas in relation to things people already understand. So people feel more confident with the new idea," James said.

"We like to share things that make us appear good rather than bad," Freida pushed on.

"Most people like to be richer, smarter, and more in shape than they actually are. So, they adopt the brands, mannerisms, and signals that convey the desired identity," James fired on.

"People sometimes adopt clothing, music, political positions, and even language to send the desired signals," Freida added.

"Sometimes people also diverge. They don't want to be misidentified. Teenagers don't want to look like their parents. Ha ha," Fatima laughed.

"Yes. At school you would have seen that jocks don't want to look like geeks," Freida laughed.

"Another thing I find that contributes to spread, is awe particularly with medical products. Awe is the sense of wonder and amazement that occurs when someone is inspired by great knowledge, beauty, or might. This works mainly in science. I have seen this at medical meetings when a new idea is presented and how everyone gathers in the breaks and discusses it and when we come home, back to work it sticks on. And bingo we have a popular product," James provided a medical perspective.

"Brand names also contribute. Wearing a top that displays the name '*Gucci*' makes it easier for people to see that you bought something expensive," Freida provided a feminine perspective.

Fatima soon realised that this topic could go on and on.

"So what food fad for us tonight?" she asked.

"I think we should try something local," Freida suggested.

"I will conform," Fatima laughed.

"I heard their *kalua pork* should be tried," James suggested.

"We'll decide when we get there," Freida left her options open.

18

Back again at Charlestown, life returned back to its mundanity.

One evening when James arrived home earlier than usual Freida was delightfully pleased.

Nevertheless she asked, "How come you are home early today?"

"It was an easy day today and I am getting more experienced at cutting corners." He smiled, quite pleased with his own pun, 'plastic surgeons cutting corners.'

"Where are the girls?" he asked.

"They are arguing about something in Fiona's room. I have been specifically requested to keep away."

"Let me go and check."

James walked up to Fiona's room and knocked.

"Anybody home?"

Silence ensued followed by laughter and Fatima answered the door.

"Hi dad," the girls chorused.

"Hi everyone. Mum said you are arguing about something. Without wanting to know what it is, I hope your argument is not about proving the other person wrong."

"No," Fiona replied.

"Yes," Faye interjected.

Fatima was quiet.

"Are you the referee Fatima?" James inquired.

Fatima smiled and nodded.

"Remember argument is essentially reasoning. That's what it is. One person makes a statement or claim for which she should provide justification. The justification can be a cause effect or it can be several independent justifications that help the claim or it can be several justifications that together help the claim. Do you girls get what I am saying?"

"Sort of," Fiona volunteered.

"I will get my head around it in time," Fatima replied as she reinforced the horizontal lines on her forehead.

"I will pick your brain later Fiona for this," Faye added.

"For evidence to your claim you can choose examples or analogies or statistics or objects or common knowledge or expert knowledge."

"I need a notebook if this is going to continue much longer," Fiona said.

"Sorry," James replied.

"You really need to be dad, especially when we were just arguing about your birthday present," Fatima helped.

"Hell, then I better be out of here or you may be biased by my opinion," James walked out after shutting the door behind him.

He joined Freida.

"What are they arguing about?" Freida inquired.

"They are deciding my birthday present."

Freida smiled.

"How nice. You know James, you and I have the best girls in the world."

"Indeed we do. We should have a son next time," James suggested.

"The body is willing but the spirit is weak," Freida replied.

James understood. Her last pregnancy with Fatima had been difficult and Freida had decided that, that would be the last one. Fatima was a breech lie and Freida had to have a caesarean section. She remembered that the post operative pain of the incision was much worse than her previous two vaginal deliveries. Her mind was firmly made up on this matter.

That night after dinner they assembled in the lounge room. This was a regular feature in the Reagan household, something he had learnt from his father, Rodney. He remembered how Rodney and Elena encouraged such discussion in their family home and guided Janet and him in many a such arguments. He and Janet had learnt a lot. His father had insisted that it showed a way for the little minds which were like sponges for knowledge. There was so much to know in so little time. Thinking back he considered himself and Janet very lucky in this regard. James had resolved he would do the same with his own children and Freida had totally co-operated. He was sure Janet would be doing the same with her imminent family. James had continued further by spending much of his free time in reading books of all genres. He was also equipped with an excellent declarative memory.

"Girls, after your earlier discourse did you settle on my present?"
"Sure did."
"It would spoil my surprise if I asked you what it is,

but no socks please."

"Noted," Fatima replied.

"After what we talked earlier it would be nice to continue on with scepticism as a topic for now. Don't you agree?" James inquired.

"That would be interesting," Freida responded.

"Scepticism is really the rigorous application of proof and reason to test the validity of a claim. The conclusions in scepticism are always provisional. And also, it is acceptable to change your mind if the evidence changes," James continued.

"So it is valid just for the time being and subject to change just like science," Faye understood.

"Yes. It allows you to change the status quo if new evidence becomes available."

"So is there life out there?" Fiona attempted to test the topic.

"The chances are high. But aliens have not visited us yet. These claims have been investigated and found to be bogus," James explained.

"So how do we decide?" Fatima used her prosecutorial acumen.

"Very good question Fatima. First decide if it is logically impossible or highly unlikely? Next see what the majority of accepted experts say on the subject. And finally is the evidence anecdotal or uncorroborated? But always, always keep an open mind," James explained.

"Did you know that psychologists are the most sceptical of all the professions?" Freida informed.

"Yes, because they deal with beliefs. In an

interesting book I read called '*Surely You're Joking, Mr. Feynman!*' this Nobel prize winner physicist provides us a principle that should serve as a guide. The principle is that you must not fool yourself and you are the easiest person to fool. Philosophers have understood for some time that humans are deeply flawed thinkers," James explained.

"I think Charles Darwin is a good example of a scientist who negotiated the essential tension between scepticism and credulity," Freida added.

"I agree. Now initially I must tell you the difference between a fact, a theory and a construct so we all start from the same page," James said.

"I know that a fact is a statement confirmed to such an extent that it would be reasonable to offer agreement," Fiona volunteered.

"Yes. That's well put, Fiona. I like it. But the agreement is only provisional. A theory must be contrasted with a construct, which is, a non-testable statement to account for a set of observations," James explained.

There was silence for a few minutes when it seemed that some were trying to digest the information so far and others were planning the next question.

"In being sceptical you must also know where to stop or you may miss out on a lot of important stuff," James went on.

"Separating the scientific wheat from the ideological chaff can be an extremely difficult task sometimes," Freida said.

"Yes that may seem the hardest part sometimes," Fiona added.

"Just because there are many things about our world that we don't fully understand doesn't mean we must deny the things we do understand in order to preserve our sense of purpose and meaning," James continued.

"We should talk about *Karl Popper* here," Freida interrupted.

"In a second," James said.

"What did you mean by theory and construct?" Fatima asked.

"Let me explain by giving you an example. If we try to explain life on earth by saying, 'god made life' then it is a construct. But if we say, 'life evolved' then it is a theory. So a theory is an explanation for some aspect of the natural world that is well supported by observed facts and tested hypotheses. Evolution is well supported by fossil evidence and by DNA evidence. A construct is not." James continued.

"Fossil records suggests that modern species have been shaped by at least five major and a dozen or more minor extinction events brought about by such disparate causes as glaciation, volcanic activity, fluctuations in sea level and asteroid impact," Freida contributed.

"As long as a given theory remains consistent with observed phenomenon and yields verifiable predictions, it must be considered a viable explanation regardless of what remains to be discovered," James explained further.

"So really in deciding these issues, we need to clarify things such as, what is the quality of the evidence and what is the background and credentials of the person making the claim," Faye wanted to clarify the essentials.

"Exactly. The probability of accepting evidence to alter a belief is provided mathematically by *Bayes' Theorem*. There can never be enough evidence to prove a hypothesis that you are unwilling to accept. This is also available in Bayes' Theorem. There are individuals who are incapable or will not change, no matter how much evidence is provided to them. If a person assigns a prior probability of zero to a hypothesis, no evidence will ever increase that probability," James continued.

"What is Bayes' theorem?" Fatima asked.

"Bayes' Theorem states that the conditional probability of an event, based on the occurrence of another event, is equal to the likelihood of the second event given the first event multiplied by the probability of the first event. Bayes theorem provides a way to calculate the probability of a hypothesis based on its prior probability, the probabilities of observing various data given the hypothesis, and the observed data itself. Sounds complicating but if you read and think about it, you will get your head around it pretty soon," James assured. Fatima was not sure but she would need to read and think about it in her own time, she thought.

"Two people might see the same evidence and come up with entirely different conclusions. They simply have different priors. A prior, or prior probability, is what you believed before you encountered new evidence," Freida added. It appeared that Freida had accessed the topic before. Being in James' company, this was not an unlikely possibility for Freida.

"I must read Bayes. It could provide more real life solutions," Fiona concluded.

"James, we should talk about Karl Popper's falsifiability now," Freida interrupted again.

"Good idea for now Freida, best you start," James said.

"The rule of falsifiability is a guarantee that if the claim is false, the evidence will prove it false; and if the claim is true, the evidence will not disprove it," Freida started.

"If the claim is invulnerable to any possible evidence then this would not mean, that the claim is true; instead it would mean that the claim is meaningless. This is the case with religions. Every true claim is falsifiable," James added.

"Any claim that could not be falsified would not be making a factual assertion. It would instead be making an emotive statement, a declaration of the way the person feels about the world," Freida attempted to explain.

"In other words, nonfalsifiable claims do communicate information, but what they describe is the person's value orientation. They communicate nothing whatsoever of a factual nature, and hence are neither true nor false," James said.

"According to Popper the distinguishing mark of science, is that it seeks to falsify, not to confirm, its hypotheses," Freida added.

"Popper believed the two standard virtues of scientific theories, explanatory power and confirmation by a large number of instances were really vices for science. Observation is really an interpretation of experience in terms of one's own theory. So fitting the data well is, thus, not the mark of a scientific theory," James went on.

"Science should make bold claims and should try to falsify these conjectures. That's what Popper is saying," Freida continued.

"Also we cannot require that a theory be rejected merely because of persistent failures of fit with the evidence. If we did that we would have little science left. Much scientific work involves trying to resolve these failures of fit," James added.

"Just like species in evolution, in the environment of science only the fittest theories will survive," Freida added.

"Rightly so," Fatima was beginning to grasp the topic.

"Because science is always decided on fact and never by fiat," James added.

"Science can only confirm or refute, it does not define or limit what is possible ahead of time. If what you believe is true, you can be assured that science will not prove you wrong. Also the scientific method knows no prejudice nor is it swayed by human sensibilities," Freida continued.

"Scientific beliefs are intrinsically amendable and thus allow for an incremental advancement of knowledge over time. Dogmatic religious beliefs offer no such flexibility and so promote stagnation of thought," James went on.

"Here belong the Muslim ayatollahs, the Catholic popes, the Jewish rabbis, the Orthodox patriarchs etcetera They are just actors acting a specific role for their own survival. I have always believed such people are not to be respected but only tolerated. And also their obedient followers who are respectful of this authority, are in same boat," Freida added.

Such topics were absolutely up Freida's and James' alleys and both of them loved discussing them with the children. The girls seemed to be enjoying it too as they listened with great interest. They admired their parents and were grateful. They felt sorry for the other children who did not have such informed parents and were not allowed to think for themselves.

"It seems to me that eventually science is not about experimentation, or evidence, or even logical inference. It is just a desire for the truth. So what would make a good scientist are interest, and the willingness to follow the interest wherever it leads to. Brightness is not necessary," Fiona surmised.

"Brightness is required to interpret the findings," Faye intercepted.

"Okay can we stop this 'all falsifiable statements are scientific but only all scientific statements are falsifiable' business now, please?" Fiona suddenly seemed to have reached the end of her tether with this stuff. When enough is enough, Fiona usually put her foot down.

"Good idea," Faye echoed.

"Just when I was beginning to not understand

anything you want to stop," Fatima joked.

"After all that discussion I would like you girls to have a very deep sense of compassion for those whose capacity for independent thought has been systematically suppressed," James advised.

"I think exactly the same, girls. That is very important to remember. Be compassionate to these people. Mostly this compassion comes with age. These older people who have done a lot of thinking in their lifetime are able to separate the wheat from the chaff quite easily. I have learnt a lot myself from Grandpa Rodney. He has my highest respect. My expectation is that the smart kids of today will become the critical thinkers of the world while their slower classmates will grow up to embrace the simplicity of dogmas and superstition," Freida added.

"Thank you Freida for those remarks about my dad. And finally a word of advice from me. It is never okay to give up on any subject you find confusing. In trying to understand complex issues, always make the time and read the same topic explained by different authors. First understand the simpler ideas. Make an active effort to clear the clutter and expose what is really important. Create questions along the way to clarify and extend your understanding. What's the real question here? The right questions will bring them out and help you see connections that otherwise would have been invisible and introduce new ideas into your head. Look back to see where the ideas came from and then look ahead to discover where those ideas may lead. A new idea is a beginning, not an end. Ideas are usually rare. Following the consequences of small ideas can result in big payoffs," James finished.

"There is another common method of proving a result that professors, teachers, and even peers will often use. I am sure you would have encountered it in class. I call it proof by humiliation. This is when a teacher fails to explain something enough, but asserts it is true. The teacher often ends by intimidating the student that he or she must be dumb not to get it. The student walks away accepting both that it is true and that he or she is incapable of understanding it. No student should allow to be academically bullied like this," Freida continued. James had discussed this before and it was good that she was reiterating, he thought.

"Then how should one deal with this situation?" Fatima inquired.

Both James and Freida were curious that Fatima wanted to know how to deal with such problems. Did she have this problem at school? Freida felt she would discuss it later with Fatima when alone.

But James wanted to nip it in the bud," What one should do is accept it as a challenge from the teacher and beat the teacher at further such duels. This requires hard work in equipping oneself with more than the teacher knows on the subject. Time and effort and determination are required with an, 'I will show you attitude'. Eventually the teacher will respect you forever after and will improve her own teaching methods."

Fatima will need to talk to Angela about integrating

her calculus attitudes along in this way.

"Time to cool off with some ice cream, girls," Freida laughed.

This invitation to dissipate was obeyed with every foot heading towards the fridge.

19

After James' undisclosed and unexpected departure, Carmen felt betrayed and was very depressed. How could I have trusted him? He appeared to be a caring person to me. I learnt a lot from him including about sex. But was it worth it? I let my guard down and shamed my entire family. Would my father have ever forgiven me if he was alive? Should I have an abortion? Could I ever trust any man again? This is my second deceiver.

Obsessed by such thoughts she tried to get through her usual mundane dailies. She often had suicidal thoughts and felt she could end all this, once and for all. Suicide was very common and easy in India particularly in young married females who did not get on well with their mothers in law. But something inside her said 'no'. Maybe it was her remnant religion or maybe it was her desire to hold on to a part of James or maybe she did not want to cause further mental damage to her mother and Cecil, her brother who would be totally devastated if she went ahead.

She decided to keep the baby as having an abortion would be the lesser of two evils for her, both physically and mentally.

Although Cecil was understanding of her situation,

her mother, Felicity stood her ground, "How could you bring this on our family? What would your father say if he was alive? Maybe God knew this and had mercy on him. I wish God would take me away too."

"I didn't know James would do this. He didn't seem like that sort of person," Carmen replied.

"Don't ever mention his name in this house again. How could you ever trust a foreigner? There are plenty of decent boys around. But not for you anymore. Why did you not talk to any of us about this before?"

"Never mind now. We will deal with this," Cecil interrupted.

"You shut up Cecil. Nobody asked you," Felicity roared back at him.

"Sorry mother," Cecil bowed out.

And such outbursts continued regularly in a progressively diminishing manner when, about a month later her mother had a change of heart possibly after her frequent daily incantations to another virgin who also fell pregnant but under greater and more mysterious circumstances. Perhaps virgins are mutually understanding.

Carmen continued to work initially until she began to show. When she was beginning to show both Carmen and her mother were slowly ostracised both by near and far relations and friends of her mother. Her mother adopted agoraphobic tendencies. Their church attendances declined. The local padres who abhorred such situations in their own parishioners were also aloof until Father Appollinarius Pereira decided to pay a visit to her mother at home.

Felicity, her mother had been a science and mathematics teacher at Gloria Convent Girls School for several years and had retired just after the death of her husband, Porfiro.

"Hello Felicity. I have not seen you at Church recently. I thought I would drop in and check how you are coping."

"Oh hello father. That is very nice of you."

"How are you?" he inquired.

She burst into tears.

"Don't worry. These things are sent to try us," he added, a very useful statement often used by the clergy to explain God's erring mind and get themselves out of providing a logical explanation.

"Never mind. God will look after you. Keep praying," he continued.

Felicity would have preferred him to keep such exegesis to his weekly sermons where she had a chance to tune off like the rest of the faithful in the pews.

Carmen continued to work at the hospital supported by her sympathetic colleagues in regard to her duties and rosters and obtained leave at about six weeks before her due date.

When she approached full term she delivered a baby boy uneventfully at Desa Maternity Hospital.

Just after delivery she held the baby for a while. He reminded her of James and of the good times. If only James could see him again? But there was no chance of that happening. Then she passed him on to her waiting mother.

The boy was unusually fair as expected and had blue eyes. Even her mother Felicity suddenly felt proud of the child in spite of her previous manifested sentiments. Felicity was actually ecstatic within but persisted with her surface cement. At that precise moment she vowed within herself that she would make the boy "the brightest and the best' in the goan community and to that end she would spare no expense. She would give science and mathematics tuitions to high school students to support her own intentions.

She advertised in the local press about her availability to tutor high schoolers and although initially she had no acceptances, the horizon changed dramatically as there was always a clear demand for private tuition in the community, in which each family sought to outdo the other particularly in their offsprings' academic achievements. This was very obvious when the mothers met at the Byculla markets for their daily bazaar purchases.

"Did your son get the clerk job into Burmah Shell Company?"

"Oh yes, he easily walked through the interview. They were very impressed with his hockey playing at St Andrews."

"And my son, Peter, you know Peter. Luckily he got into the priesthood. He will be minding the gates when St Peter retires, he says."

"And me, did you know my son John, who is a Marist priest is one of only five priests from all over the world who has been selected by the pope to come to Rome to help him? But our John has decided not to go." Of course John did not want to go because there was no substance in the story. And be it known thus, all ye present here, John is not an ordinary garden variety priest. He has refused the pope.

Each mother at the market knew that all these stories were made up to impress the other mothers and there was absolutely no truth in any, to which they often made generous contributions themselves. As a result the stories were not usually promulgated beyond the narrator by the audience.

The priests at Gloria Church refused to baptise Carmen's child with the usual expected exclamations, "It is not in my hands. The cardinal has to authorise it." When this avenue was chased, "The pope has to authorise it," followed. Carmen understood the lackey clergy attitude. She was reminded of the validity of James' discourses.

In all this turmoil, the boy, Rowan DeCruz was growing up and was admitted at four years of age to Holy Cross School across the road where they lived. Under the tutelage of his grandmother the boy excelled in his studies and was soon the envy of his fellow students as he was far advanced in his knowledge.

He was slowly growing to be taller than his mother and acquired a disgusting habit of rolling his tongue when he spoke. His grandmother was importunate in her admonitions of the habit and warned him routinely that that it would not stand him in good stead in decent company. Rowan tried very hard to please her but was mostly not successful.

The children at school mocked him calling him a parsi and rolling their tongue to utter "*bhavaji kon che*", (parsi for "brother, who is there?") and tried to annoy him thus. However the boy had learnt how not to be upset from his grandmother's instructions and smiled his way through disarming their attempts. Some children got frustrated and may even have resorted to violence but refrained after pre-empting the outcome of such an encounter in view of Rowan's height and build.

Days gave way to years and Rowan was admitted to St Xavier's High School at Dhobitalao. Rowan excelled in English, Science and Mathematics in the School certificate examination. He did biology at St Xavier's College and was later admitted to Grant Medical College at JJ Hospital for graduate medical studies.

His days at medical school were very enjoyable. For once he was unsupervised and felt really free. In medical school it was rumoured that he was of parsi lineage with a plausible parsi mother. Other details were not required by fellow students at this stage of teenage maturity.

Amusement and pranks were provided by some jovial fellow students and also even by some of the teachers at medical school. The junior teachers particularly, also understood the stress of medical studies as some of them were pursuing higher qualifications themselves.

The lecture theatres were also being used by the

local pigeons as boarding houses. Attempting to extract some humour out of the situation one student opened an umbrella above his head in the lecture theatre one day. The fellow students looked forward to an amusing outcome in the situation.

However the middle aged lecturer was not amused, "Mr Ginde, please shut your umbrella."

"Sir, I have a new shirt. I am just protecting it just in case the pigeons have diarrhoea."

The student audience roared with laughter.

"You know that opening an umbrella indoors brings bad luck."

The umbrella went shut immediately. No one can afford bad luck on the Indian subcontinent and particularly not in an Indian medical school.

At another time, a lady student entered the physiology lecture class well beyond the starting time. All eyes turned on her as she uttered sheepishly, "Sorry I am late today sir, I overslept at home."

"What! I can't believe that. Are you implying that you sleep at home as well as here?" the lecturer responded. A large laughter applause was provided by the other students.

As usual in medical school scenarios there is always at least one very studious student. Sudhir, with an apparent associated 'looking for love' schedule on his agenda provided this role. It was thought that the thickness of the lenses in his spectacles bore evidence to the long hours he had spent in their usage. It was rumoured that he attempted to leave himself knowledgeable to impress the women students. However the other male students including Rowan took every opportunity to debunk and humiliate his efforts publicly, often returning Sudhir for a further re- read of the books. Sudhir thus usually bore the major brunt of the mockery available in the vicinity.

One day Sudhir arrived in a red Fiat motor car. The car provided enough material to provoke the humour hormones of those assembled around.
"Sudhir your car is great."
"Thank you."
"I love that in your car everything makes a noise except the horn."

Sudhir was also preyed upon at the compulsory national service training sessions every Wednesday evening. At the firing range the students humoured that with his spectacle lens' thickness, when Sudhir fired the rifle, the safest place to be was on the target itself.

Another day Sudhir arrived with a three legged dog in his car. Some girls hovered around the dog showering verbal sympathy.
"What's his name?"
"Lucky"
"What happened to his leg?"
"He had an accident"
"Did you name him 'Lucky' before or after the accident?"

After a while Sudhir acquired immunity to the remarks and developed the 'deaf ear syndrome', wherein one only smiles and does not provide any further material for fuel, with smarter counter remarks. The mockers looked for new targets to keep the humour ball rolling. Rowan with his tongue rolling was himself the subject of laughter on several occasions. However by now he had learnt how to handle the situation without post incident perturbation.

The students also often mimicked and mocked the obsessive teachers in their absence, provoking more laughs. Rowan enjoyed it all and looked forward to every single day at medical school.

One season, the rain god was admiring its own prowess at being able to humiliate the sun at this time of the year causing gross havoc and had continued to persist thus for a few days. The physiology lecture was due to start soon. The silence was deafening. The students equipped with closed umbrellas and recent smiles appeared to be recovering from a humorous episode, as the professor of physiology entered and was about to deliver his lecture. As he was in the process of defumigating his cigar he noted the fresh wet footmarks on the desks and benches and inquired, "Who has been walking on the furniture with dirty shoes?"

Everyone was quiet.

"It is obvious that this person has not been brought up to respect other people's property", the professor went on. "Who was it? Own up or there will be serious consequences."

Everyone was quiet.

Perhaps to avoid further derogation of his own parents, a hand shot up, "It was me," the professor's own son in the audience admitted.

The professor appeared visibly perturbed. He was not prepared for this," Come and see me immediately after this lecture."

What transpired between them later was not available for public knowledge.

Initially some parsi girls, in search of amorous consequences attempted to gain Rowan's attention. On realising he was not of a parsi timbre they soon retracted and let it be known around that he was a goan. The goan army of three girls descended on him next but with no success. These particular goan girls, all being of an androgynous flowering, lowered his testosterone levels to subnormal levels. The other three goan boys in his year at the medical school were also similarly influenced hormonally by these girls.

Another goan student, Michael attempted to introduce Rowan to smoking. However, Rowan did not find the experience very pleasing. Michael told him he should try it again. Rowan was not convinced and had made up his mind to forfeit any further advice from Michael along these lines.

That evening his grandmother, Felicity smelled the smoke in his breath. Disaster. He should have stayed out longer or gone to the movies. It was too late.

"Have you been smoking Rowan?"

"Yes a friend pushed me to."

"A friend? Do you call that a friend?"

"I promise not to do it again."

Felicity knew when her battle was won and when to

drop her arms.

Michael also loved the hopelessly inebriate state provided by alcohol at parties. Rowan realised that Michael's company would not help him realise his own ambitions and soon drifted away from him, avoiding Michael at every turn. Although upset, Michael on his part understood Rowan's wishes and cooperated.

Often, Rowan would accompany Vasco, another goan student to lunch across the road to a goan restaurant. *Pork vindaloo* with rice were Rowan's favourite dishes. Pork vindaloo is a pungent red chilly dish with garlic and vinegar. The waiters who knew him at the goan restaurant often placed his standing order when they saw him arriving at the door. Rowan appreciated this service, as it saved him time in getting back to his scheduled presences across the road.

Some students did not survive the rigors of the study required to please the examiner doctors, who stressed heavily on the ability of the students to memorise, to ensure a pass. Also it was well known that some of the teachers were ardent supporters of the nepotistic school of student examination. The beneficiaries also were well known.

Further years in medical school were not as disruptive. This was understandable considering the increasing maturity with time, among the students and the academic weeding and pruning in the initial couple of years.

Mention must be made of the obstetric term which was despised by Rowan who did not like the smell of the *liquor amnii* wafting in the ward. He avoided the obstetric ward totally, in spite of having to assist in at least twenty mandatory deliveries as per the regulations. In this regard he was aided by the nurses who loved him and his smiles, and provided the necessary signatures for his log book without requiring his actual physical presence.

In all this, Rowan often aided by his grandmother's frequent admonitions, kept his committed mission going. He had decided to become a plastic surgeon like his deceased father. He now kept mainly to himself and spent any free time he had, studying. Carmen and his grandmother who had now withdrawn out of their self-inflicted mental confinements would sometimes entice him to accompany them for a walk at Mahim Beach. Mahim Beach is located to the north of Byculla and they got there by taxi. During such times Rowan often inquired about his dad and the answers were only provided by Carmen. Rowan was much disturbed that he never got to meet his dad. The only consolation provided was by his grandmother, "God works in mysterious ways" and Rowan accepted that as an explanation of his predicament.

He was determined to excel in his studies and after graduation completed the postgraduate Master of Surgery studies in plastic surgery. He stood first at the examination amongst fourteen other candidates.

He was also excellent in his operative skills as a surgeon and his consultants were very proud of him and trusted his decisions completely.

20

Rowan had applied for a training fellowship overseas and was delighted to be informed of a position available at Newcastle Australia. He jumped at the opportunity and applied immediately. About two months later he received a reply that the position would be available provided he passed the American Educational Certificate for Foreign Medical Graduates exam abbreviated to ECFMG and an English language test. This was no problem as he had already passed the American exam in readiness for a possible appointment in America. And English was his quasi mother tongue. The Australian position was more appealing with residence facilities and board provided.

About a month later he received a reply confirming his appointment as a fellow.

Another month later in December he was at Sydney airport amazed at the slow pace of life compared to Bombay. Nowhere was the heat or the noise of Bombay. In fact he felt bearably cold and wished for more layers of clothing. But that will have to wait.

He stayed the night at the YMCA hostel in Sydney and took the early train to Newcastle on the next morning. The train ride took about three hours. The few passengers in the train were mainly females causing some disharmony in his hormones and prompting erections which he was able to mentally suppress. He had been used to this plight with girls in Bombay and suppression was almost an instinct and habit now with him.

He presented himself to the medical superintendent on arrival at the hospital. The medical superintendent was a middle aged gentleman with a sympathetic smile who seemed to understand the problems of immigrant doctors. He attempted to simplify his English for Rowan, so that he would not be humiliated. However he was soon surprised by Rowan's command of the language.

"Where did you learn such good English?" he inquired.

"English is my mother tongue. We speak English at home," he responded.

"That is really very interesting. Most of the Indian residents we have here struggle with even the English of their own names, although they have all passed the English language test. We had an interesting one called Manesh who insisted on being called Hamish. Rather odd."

Later the medical superintendent walked him to his allocated quarters.

The shower and toilet facilities were common with the other residents. Rowan was very much pleased with the available accommodation. Having explained to him the essentials including the availability of meals at the hospital canteen, the medical superintendent requested him to report to the outpatients department on the next day and left him.

Rowan decided to explore the hospital initially and then the surrounds. The hospital had two buildings, both of entirely separate eras. The outpatients department was in the older section and the in-patient wards were in the newer building. His accommodation was in the older building. Later he explored the nearby streets around using the hospital as a marker, just like a child venturing forward on its own and always looking back and making sure a parent is visible.

Rowan saw James his supervising consultant, in the outpatients department the next morning. James was conveying some instructions to a nurse.

"Good morning sir, I am Rowan DeCruz, your new fellow," Rowan introduced himself attempting to keep his tongue rolling under control, as per his grandmother's instructions.

James looked at him, "Welcome Rowan. We have been expecting you. We are a busy lot here as you will soon find out. I hope you enjoy your stay here with us," James replied also rolling his tongue.

Rowan was as tall as James.

"I am sure I will sir," Rowan replied.

During this encounter, James did notice that Rowan had a habit of rolling his tongue. He was not concerned and it did not matter to him. After all he rolled his own tongue too, he thought. James showed him around the hospital and introduced him to the relevant staff.

He told him the various responsibilities that he would be liable for. Rowan listened very carefully.

His duties were similar to that of the registrar, who would share the on call duty with him on alternate weeks. He was required to do outpatients, some operating, teaching and some research work.

"Have you any particular research project in mind Rowan that you wish to pursue here?" James inquired.

"I am interested in keloid scarring sir," he replied.

"Fortunately for us we do not have much keloid scarring here. But I saw some cases in the Marshall Islands when I went there. But we have a lot of melanoma here, if that interests you."

Rowan had not heard of the Marshall Islands. He preferred not to expose his ignorance and jettisoned any thoughts in his mind of inquiring further on the matter. He would check about the Marshall Islands himself later tonight. James felt that Rowan would be aware of the Marshall Islands with all its bombing history.

"Yes sir. But I need to read a bit more about melanoma," Rowan replied rolling his tongue. James was generally pleased with Rowan's demeanour and most of all, with his English skill. He also had encountered Indian residents before that stressed him even with the English of their own names! He remembered Chetan, a resident he had a couple of years ago who insisted on being called Ethan.

Rowan got along well with all the staff and was liked by all. He was always very pleasant, polite and obliging. The nurses soon realised that Rowan was the easiest to manipulate and called on him to get any medical work done, from signing a prescription to setting up an intravenous drip at odd hours. He was the easiest non-complaining doctor to call upon, even when he was not on call. He was very punctual in all his assignments and left only after all the work was fully done.

One day when James was operating, the theatre nurse Stella, who was assisting said to him, "James, your fellow Rowan, tries so hard to imitate you in every way. I have watched him operating and he has operating movements just like yours. He is no longer himself, whatever that was. It is not healthy for him to idolise you so much."

"All plastic surgeons have the same characteristic operating movements. We are all trained to be like that you know," James replied.
"I know, but he is too much like you. I would have thought he is your younger brother but I know you do not have a younger brother," she responded.

James did not want to pursue the matter any further, as it was not a bother to him and he was at this moment really occupied by the bleeder that he was trying stop. Seeing so, the nurse relinquished her probing.
"Cautery please."

When he had finished and was on his way to the change room, the thought reappeared to him. Could he be Carmen's son? No, it is not possible. India has millions of people. The chances are remote. It is most unlikely.

He went to the ward to check on his postoperative patients. Rowan was there. He looked at him more closely. No, not possible.

Rowan approached him, "Good evening sir, I have checked on all the patients and all is well."

"Thank you Rowan. You have a good evening too."

On his way to the car, he decided not to let such thoughts bother him again. But could he really?

The next day he saw Rowan in the outpatients department. Rowan was busy attending to a waiting patient.

"Good morning sir," Rowan said on seeing James.

"Good morning Rowan. How are you?" James replied.

"Very good sir," Rowan responded rolling his tongue.

"What have you got there?" James inquired.

"Just a fractured zygoma with visible displacement. It should be easy to fix. I will try and find a time in theatre. The patient is fasting. I can manage."

"I'm sure you will do a good job," James replied consciously resisting his own tongue movements.

"However before you go I would like you see a patient in the ward. He came in last night with a grade four facial palsy. His general practitioner had him on steroids and acyclovir. His eye closure is bad and the eye is desiccating in spite of the lubricating drops. The ENTs want us to consider putting a stitch on the lids.

"Fine, can we go see him?"

"Sure sir. Dana can you get them to page me when they find a time in theatre," Rowan said to the nurse who was helping him.

"Yes doctor." She responded.

As James and Rowan progressed toward the new building the sun was very bright. As soon as they stood in its light both of them had a bad sneezing fit.

"The sun always gets me. It seems you have a similar problem sir," Rowan began.

"Yes, it does get me sometimes. Our Australian sun is very strong. We have a very high incidence of skin cancer."

Our Indian sun is no less sir. But skin cancer rates are not high. Oral cancer is very high due to the betel nut chewing," Rowan explained.

James knew about the betel nut problem in Bombay. He remembered hearing that from Dr. Bhatt and wondered how Dr.Bhatt would have responded to his disappearance from JJ Hospital all those years ago when James had invited him to come to Australia. Dr. Bhatt would be happy he did not take up James' offer seriously. James could not be trusted.

As they walked across towards the wards, James was feeling uncomfortable with his thoughts. Could this Rowan be is son? How odd would that be? If he is, how would he deal with it in his present environment? What will Freida say? What would his daughters think of their dad? He needed more information about Rowan and his family. But how? Without causing suspicion in other minds? He needed to talk to Rowan. He could ask him for a drink. What if he did not drink? Nevertheless he should try.

"Rowan do you drink alcohol?"

"Of course I do sir. I am a goan Indian. Goans have a special reputation for drinking alcohol."

The word goan is exactly what James did not want to hear and with his surname being DeCruz, the penny had finally dropped for James. This could be his own son. Serendipity at its worst. There was no way out of this. He wished this chapter had not included him.

"Would you like to join me for a drink this evening at Fannys pub at the corner?" James asked.

Rowan could not believe his ears. The boss asking him to join for a drink? Alcohol? An almost unheard event from where he came from, in Bombay. He thought that Dr Firoze Mehta, his consultant in JJ Hospital in Bombay would rather be dead than eat or drink with his residents. The bosses in Bombay considered themselves to be deities and the subordinates were mere mortals who in time would become deities if they possessed the necessary nepotistic connections. Goans being Christians did not feature much in this hierarchy.

Or maybe James just wanted to talk about his progress at work. He had no choice but to accept.

"I would very much like to, sir," Rowan accepted.

"I will see you there at six o'clock this evening, all being well. I have a small private list this afternoon. Not much, just some lumps and bumps."

"Most certainly sir, I will meet you there."

As they went into the ward, Rowan escorted James to bed number eleven. The patient was asleep.

"Don't wake him up. You know what to do."

"Surely sir. It is not a problem."

"I will see you later," James walked away.

"Definitely sir."

James liked Rowan. He was such a pleasant young man. If he was not related he would not have minded him as his son in law. But as a son, no, he did not need a son right now under the prevailing circumstances.

Rowan was able to fit the fractured zygoma and the eyelid suture at the end of the dental list to finish in ample time to meet James.

When he had finished in the theatre he ran up to his room and hurriedly shaved and showered. He pampered his integument with a sandalwood deodorant before wearing a light cerulean blue shirt and navy blue pants. He wore an orange tie to match.

Fannys was within walking distance from the hospital and on a slightly downward slope. He found the walk conducive to his prevailing mood. He could almost burst into a song. But which song? *I could have danced all night?*

He arrived at five thirty five and was pleased with his ambulatory effort. He felt it was almost tantamount to his own thoughts of dancing. Should he wait outside or go in? What if James is inside? He went in and had a quick look. No definitely, he is not inside. He came outside and stood by the door.

He watched the passers-by and noted that some

young men were returning back from a swim, with towels still tied round their waist and their upper torso exposed. There were also some loud girls with swimwear and towels and their upper torso selectively unexposed.

James arrived at last more than several minutes late.

"Sorry I am a bit late. One four flap z-plasty took a bit longer than I expected. Couldn't get the fit right for a while."

"No problem sir," Rowan responded.

"Rowan, I would appreciate if you don't call me sir this evening."

"Understood." Perhaps he did not like to be addressed as 'sir' in public places, Rowan thought.

"Let's go in and sit down. I have been standing all afternoon."

"You lead the way. I have not been here before."

"Okay, follow me."

Rowan rolled his tongue and was just about to "sir" him when he remembered his recent instructions.

"Let's sit down here," James said, pointing to an unoccupied table by the window.

"Okay."

They sat at the table. It was a bit warm inside and both of them were grateful for the minimal current of air that managed to be misled within, from outside. Rowan was regretting his decision to wear a tie.

"What will you drink Rowan?"

"Just a beer, thank you."

"Any particular brand?"

"No, any will do. But can I please pay?" Rowan inquired.

"Tonight is my shout Rowan. You can pay another time."

Another time? The weight of going through another time for a repeat of this occasion was enough to shut up Rowan momentarily.

James went off to the bar and came back with two full beer glasses and placed them on the table.

He lifted one and held it towards Rowan, "Cheers."

Rowan reciprocated with the other glass.

Both had a mouthful and put the glasses down.

"I needed that drink. How was your day Rowan? Do you like it at the hospital?" James asked.

"Very much so."

"Tell me something about yourself Rowan."

"What would you like to know?"

"I find your English is very good and your surgical skill is brilliant. I am curious to know about your family and upbringing and where you trained and all that. Please start."

"Well, I am from Byculla in Bombay and I went to Grant Medical College and JJ Hospital."

The familiarity of the names was bothering James very much now. He was almost sure of what was coming. Nevertheless he was hopeful.

"What do your parents do?"

"My mother was a nurse at JJ Hospital and my father died in a plane crash before I was born. My grandmother who was a retired school teacher looked after me mainly."

James was now absolutely sure that Rowan was his son. Suddenly he felt proud that Rowan was his son. He had three daughters, Fiona the eldest was twenty five and was a physiotherapist, Fatima was twenty and a speech therapist and Felicity the youngest was fifteen and still at school.

"That is interesting because here in Australia, grandmothers have an unwelcome role."

"Not so in India. Every relation has a role, whether welcome or unwelcome," Rowan produced an efforted laugh.

"How is your mother? Does she write to you often?"

"Yes, very very often. Last week I received two letters from her. I often don't get time to write back as quickly."

"No, you should write to her as often as possible. Will you have something to eat?"

"No, I will eat later in the hospital canteen."

"Hospital food, don't you get fed up of it?"

"No I like it. The hospital is very kind to give it to me."

James realised the irony of his own remarks within the Indian context.

"I will get some pizzas. Which one would you like? Here's the menu," James handed it to him.

Rowan did not make any effort to look at the menu. This was not a time to make any mistakes, "I will have whichever one you are having."

"Two Margheritas then."

"Fine," Rowan replied hoping his response was appropriate.

James went off to order and pay and returned back to the table. On his return, he sat quietly lost in thought. The pizzas arrived in a short while.

As they were consuming the pizzas, James was still lost in thought and very pensive. How could he have behaved like that to Carmen and Rowan? There is no way he could make up to Carmen. Perhaps he could usurp Rowan into his schedule if he confessed to Freida. How would Freida take it if she knew his past? How would the girls respond if they knew what he had done?

Noting James' taciturnity Rowan surmised he may have said something to upset James, but he was not sure.

James wanted to find out more about Carmen to plan his further moves and seek a way out.

"I am interested to know more about you Rowan."

The normally reticent James was now talking more than usual.

"Really."

"Tell me about more about your parents."

"As I mentioned before my father was a plastic surgeon. I decided to be a plastic surgeon to be more like him for my mother. That's the main reason I became a plastic surgeon."

"What's your father's name?"

"My father died before I was born," tears welled in Rowan's eyes.

"And your mother?"

"She was a nurse at JJ Hospital. She does not work anymore"

"So what does she do now?"

"She cries. I think she misses my dad. She goes to church very often. In fact most of the time. She prays to God to take her away too so she can be with dad."

James' heart was bleeding hard. He wanted to bury his head in the ground and disappear forever. How could he have done this?

Should he stop questioning Rowan now? No. This may be the only chance he may get to talk to Rowan very privately.

"Where does your mother live?"

"At Byculla. When my grandmother died she left the house for her."

James was firmly determined to see Carmen again. But how? He must look for a way somehow. Carmen was beginning to hurt him very much now.

21

After Rowan left for Australia, Carmen was very lonely and spent most of her time in crying and in prayer. She did not go out at all and spent time remembering her demised mother with whom she had finally cemented a firm relationship aided by Rowan's academic successes.

Felicity, her mother died of breast cancer. She had ignored, for quite some time the left breast nipple pus discharge she had, hoping it would abate soon. This was later accompanied by pain and blood discharge. She was feeling constantly tired and nauseated and was losing her appetite. She spent a significant amount of time in bed often claiming there was nothing wrong with her. Carmen could see that she was losing weight and implored her regularly to come with her to see Dr. Lima, the family doctor. By the time she finally decided to see Dr. Lima she had secondaries in her lymph nodes and spine and walked with a slight limp.

Soon the cancer was in her lungs and caused her shortness of breathing. She died within six months of seeing the doctor. Carmen was devastated. She wrote to let Rowan know.

After her mother's death and in Rowan's absence, Carmen's anxiety and grief took control and she was often times totally engrossed in severe crying episodes. Goan women never run out of tears and Carmen was reared and bred to do so. Tales of sadness abounded in Byculla and spiced with the particularly distinctive flavour available in the myths of Catholicism and particularly prompted by the ubiquitous depictions of the ever suffering mother of Jesus, Mary and the crucifixion, these provide a readymade provocation for lacrimal stimulation for goan women. There are also ample opportunities available for rehearsal in goan company, as every story that is verbally narrated or experienced or imagined must have always have a sad ending.

Her brother Cecil visited her often and sometimes times with his wife and children. Sometimes he brought her some food from the local restaurants and at other times, food cooked by his wife Esther, who was very fond of Carmen.

Carmen always looked forward to any mail from Rowan. Rowan was dejected on hearing the news of Felicity's death. In his letter, Rowan promised Carmen a trip to Australia as soon as he could manage. She was otherwise pleased that he had a good boss who liked him.

One day as she was scanning the local papers she was attracted to an advertisement which offered higher education. The institution was located at Churchgate and offered flexible hours. Rather than drift rudderless, she decided she would do a degree in psychology and may be learn to deal at least with her own demons.

She got up early the next day and made her way to Kishinchand Chellaram College, commonly known as KC College which was located near the Churchgate railway station. The building was impressive and Carmen ventured inside to investigate. The young adolescent students roamed around like ants, unengrossed by the surrounds and as if searching for an opening to the outside where they may fulfil their imminent gustatory and other quasi romantic desires.

In the College office, the desk was manned or rather unmanned by two women who were permanently engrossed in conversation, providing narratives to each other in measured instalments with intervals for questions. Carmen managed to gain their attention and enrolled for an Arts degree with Indian history as subsidiary and psychology as major. The course was to begin in a few days. She was able to attend the morning sessions. Carmen was quite excited at this opportunity.

The Indian history course dealt with early Indus Valley civilisation which flourished from about 2600 to 1900 BC. This civilisation included cities such as Harappa, and Mohenjo-daro. It was interesting to note that Alexander the Great came up to the north of India in his warring efforts. Apparently he was under the impression that the world ended beyond India and he possibly had no intentions of falling off the map with his armies. The in-migration of Arian or Indo-European peoples, settled down into a major empire in the 4th century BC, as the Mauryan Empire and, at the end of the classical period was followed by the

Gupta Empire. Others like, the Mughal Empire, the Maratha Empire and British Empire followed, finally giving way to the Indian Independence in 1947. Although she had had glimpses of this history in school this was her chance to usurp the details.

In psychology she was keen to learn about Sigmund Freud and *id, ego* and *superego* and his dream theories and psychoanalysis. She was impressed by Skinner and his theories of conditioned learning. She tried to reconcile Piaget's theory with Rowan's development as an infant and had many pleasant moments reminiscing.

Why had she not thought of doing this degree several years ago? It gave her a new perspective on life.

Often as she walked on the main street and especially when she walked past Gaylords restaurant she remembered James, sometimes with love but mostly with hatred.

The course proceeded eventfully with Carmen topping the class in every exam much to the envy of her younger colleagues who nicknamed her "old lady" to equilibrate their jealousy. However her Parsi lecturers who were mainly female, admired and complimented her both in in class and outside.

Eventually Carmen claimed the degree with first class honours and was quite pleased with herself. Her mother would definitely have been proud of her if she was alive. Life is not fair. She had worked it well by now. God only looks after those who look after themselves. How true! So really is there a need for a god? To help whom? Doubts attempted to creep in.

She went out for a meal with Cecil and his wife and their two boys, that night at a local restaurant to celebrate her achievement. The many hours of hard study were finally vindicated.

"I am very proud of you Carmen," Cecil complimented her.

"Yes I take my hat off to you Carmen. You have done very well," Esther, Cecil's wife added.

"Thank you."

"How is Rowan going in Australia?" Cecil wanted to know.

"Very good. He has an excellent boss."

"You have a very bright boy there, Carmen. I think he has a great future when he comes back here," Esther added further.

"Only God knows. I pray he does not fall for an Australian girl and then he won't come back as happened to Maggie's son when he went to America."

"What has to happen will happen Carmen. No point in worrying," Cecil consoled.

They enjoyed the meal and Cecil paid.

Next morning she received a message from the psychology professor to consider joining the psychology staff of KC College which opportunity she gladly accepted. This called for another celebration. She invited Cecil and his family again. This time she would pay.

Carmen was assigned to teach abnormal and forensic psychology initially, both subtopics she thoroughly enjoyed. Finally life was beginning to be good for her, she thought.

Her lectures were scheduled for the weekday mornings which implied being at the college staff room by 7.00 am. Depending on the level of individual interest, the students appeared in instalments for the lecture after 7.30 am. Initial daily higher attendances were soon followed by lower attendances, as friendships were made and student mutual interests outside the classroom gained priority.

As she explored the abnormal psychology subject further for her teaching purposes, she was beginning to understand her own self very much better. She remembered her own times, when she had fallen into those great deep wells of depression and how she could have helped herself and her mother if only she had known better then. She was appalled and embarrassed when she remembered her own social withdrawals and feelings of guilt, her extreme mood changes, tantrums and outbursts in those days! Her crying episodes, her feelings of tiredness, low energy and problems with sleeping finally had a real meaning. Just thinking about it now she was beginning to feel guilty again. Giving a damn was perhaps the right thing to do.

This advice smelled of James and he was another deep well for her, to be avoided too.

She was also beginning to realise that religion along

with all its rituals to be followed was basically a human obsessive-compulsive disorder.

Her explorations into forensic psychology for the teaching purposes carried her into a different realm. Sometimes just reading about the cases interfered with her sleep. She could never ever be a practising forensic psychologist she thought. However she enjoyed teaching the subject.

One day in the corridor, as luck would have it, the senior forensic professor, Mrs Freny Mistry who had a private forensic practice in the Fort area of the city approached her. Mrs Mistry was looking for someone to replace her as an expert witness in an impending case. Mrs Mistry wanted to go to Canada to help her daughter who was due to go into labour soon. The 29 year old respondent, Mr Shah in the trial was clearly an untreated schizophrenic who had murdered his neighbour's wife who, Mr Shah felt was reading his thoughts and monitoring him. Mrs. Freny informed Carmen that her only obligation was to provide an unbiased opinion so that justice was could be administered.

Carmen was apprehensive and requested time to consider.

"I'm counting on you Carmen."

"You know I have never done this before."

"Believe me. It is not difficult. I have all the details of this case. But it would be good to examine the respondent yourself with his solicitor, Mr. Solanki. I can arrange that for you. "

On the next day, in the staff room, Carmen advised

Mrs Freny Mistry to go ahead and book her ticket to Canada.

The prosecuting barrister guessed that Carmen was a rookie in this game. He kept his questions simple.

As expected the defendant was released on grounds of insanity with a compulsory medical treatment order. Carmen was relieved her work was done. She resolved she would never allow herself to be put into this position again. She herself needed a holiday now.

On her way home from court she decided that she would take a single week holiday to her family home in Goa. She had earned it, she thought. As a child, going to Goa was an obligation in the school holidays that she had always looked forward to. Annually, her parents, Cecil and herself would board the train for the journey to Margao, Goa. Porfiro, her father was an employee with the Western Railway. He was responsible for claiming the space for the family on this Central Railway train departing from Queen Victoria Train terminus. With verbal and physical threats to fellow passengers, his efforts procured sufficient space to allow basic respiratory effort for the family, for the journey. Any hiatus noted by fellow passengers in the vicinity was soon occupied by some part of their own self anatomy. Felicity provided the required prepacked subsidence replenishments for the required twenty four hours. Along the way at every stop, they had to contend with experienced hawkers who attempted to reduce every passenger's monetary advantage to their own benefit often with an added bonus of post journey diarrhoea.

This time however, she would fly in comfort on an Air India plane from Santa Cruz domestic airport. She wrote a letter to Rowan exposing her excitement.

On the plane trip her thoughts retracted to her recent court appearance. In spite of all the song and dance, the courts do not really administer justice in the true sense of the word. They merely try to settle a dispute between two parties in favour of one or the other. The objective is just to settle the dispute by any means. This does not imply that the winning party is not guilty. That did bother her. The newspaper reporters misunderstand it as true justice which, it is then publicly promulgated as such. The law understands that it is better to set a criminal free rather then incarcerate an innocent person.

The family home was at Milhamvaddo, Cuncolim, Salcette Goa. Her mother, Felicity used to leave the house key with the Hindu neighbours next door with instructions for repairs and then provided the required reimbursements. The arrangements had remained the same, except that Cecil managed it now.

Nothing had changed in Cuncolim since she last visited so acclimatisation was not on her agenda. Even the doctor's pharmacy had not demanded new paint.

She decided to attend mass at Our Lady of Health Church at Milhamvaddo next morning. She had gratitude to convey.

She arrived a bit early at the old familiar church which incidentally had been blessed with a fresh coat of paint. She decided to convey her gratitude by imparting a hundred rupees, when the usual plate was passed around. She went in and occupied a place in one of the back pews. The church was fairly vacant except for some elderly people, who possibly used it as St. Peter's waiting room.

Some notes of solemn music were released and the priest choreographed his dance in. Carmen could not believe her eyes. It was Joseph Carvalho. His horizontal dimensions had increased grossly with his abdominal integument seeking to aid the gravitational forces and asymmetric ageometric lines occupied his face twice over. How lucky she was to have escaped him, she thought.

Father Joseph Carvalho usually took a visual note of his attendees to obtain some idea of the impending plate grossage to manage his cash flow. He recognised her in a back pew. A pang ran into his heart. He felt ashamed. He had left for the priesthood one day without even telling her. There was no time for thoughts now. He had to continue with the mass. He only hoped she would not come up for communion.

Carmen left early to avoid him. She had enough catholic dirty linen herself she could not wash in public.

Later in the afternoon there was a knock on her

front door. She opened the door and it was Father Carvalho. He reeked of alcohol.

"Come in Father."

"Thank you my girl. How are you?"

"I am well Father."

After the preliminaries to include current positions were exchanged, Father Joseph Carvalho ventured, "I had always wanted to come and see you. I have wanted to do this for a very long time. But by the grace of God this has happened now."

There was silence. Carmen had no words to say.

Father Joseph continued, "I owe you the greatest apology ever. When I joined we were specifically instructed not to see any girl friends in case that may cause us to change our minds. With my family circumstances I had no choice but to join. My mother was adamant and so was my father. But I am beginning to recognise my fallacy now. But it is too late. With all my clergical degrees, even some from the overseas higher catholic institutions, my employability in the real outside world is nil. I can only be employed by the church institutions."

Carmen was only hoping he would not propose to her. There was no way she would fall this time.

She felt like telling him to pray but that would be ironical.

"I'm sorry to hear that."

"Can you forgive me?"

"Don't you ever worry about it. I am fine."

"You must understand that life in the priesthood is

very lonely. There is no physical or emotional intimacy. Even if you decide to live celibate, your sexuality is still there. Some of us have clandestine affairs which we can pick up in the confessionals. Sometimes one has to resort to alcohol."

Carmen did not like the route this conversation was taking. What to do now?

"I am very sorry for you Father. Pray to God and he will look after you."

She had struck the right note. Father Joseph himself had used this line many a time in his parish at funerals to allay grieving widows concerned about feeding their many children. Realising there was no opening here of any kind, "Yes, I must go now. I have work to do."

"Goodbye Father."

She was glad to see the soutaned alcoholic go.

She would be avoiding that church on this holiday.

In fact she would be avoiding all churches and frocked clergy on this holiday.

Next day she took the bus to Margao. Securing a seat in competition with the other semi clad humans, oinking pigs and clucking poultry was quite a feat. The buses had no scheduled time of departure and the time was decided when the bus reached the maximum capacity. The wooden seats, allowed the locally grown groins to take note of every dip on the road and even consider an evolutionary change in the gluteal region in the future, under the circumstances.

She busied herself around in Margao trying to find

something to buy. Considering she had to keep in with the weight restrictions on luggage in the plane, her choices were very limited. She would like to buy some gifts for Cecil and his family.

She had *pork sorpotel* and *shark ambot tik* rice aided by a Kingfisher beer for lunch at Longuinhos restaurant situated at the crossroads. Sorpotel is a tangy and spicy meat curry introduced by the Portuguese. Shark ambot tik is made from small baby sharks with a cartilaginous spine and a particular spice combination and tomato puree which provides an acid flavour.

She brought some novels from a bookshop and then proceeded to the bus stop for a bus back to Cuncolim. Somehow there were no pigs or poultry to compete with, on the way back. Carmen's attention to the vibrating wooden seats was now forcibly commanded by the ensuing discomfort. The road was more heavily cratered than Jupiter's moon, Callisto.

She was relieved when her destination was announced but was not sure if a mobility issue might be waiting for her as she quickly jumped off the bus, taking her chances.

To her surprise, she was able land and to walk home without great difficulty.

The novels helped her erase the residual time of her holiday.

For some time she had been looking for a topic for a research project. On the way back on the plane it struck her that she had read somewhere that only two per cent of catholic priests are celibate. Yes, it was *Richard Sipe*, she remembered, the monk priest and psychotherapist who wrote that. She could use this information either in abnormal psychology or even in forensic psychology. She needed time to dissect the thought further. She was hoping to write a paper soon on the subject.

22

The music was blaring on Hunter Street in Newcastle city. It was Christmastime. David Jones, the city's major department store, portrayed the Christmas scenes and the Santa Claus myths in full glory, with life size statues in its display windows. Rudolph, the red nosed reindeer was repeatedly performing some predetermined movements which delighted some of the locally employed adult passers-by. They would spend a considerable amount of time frozen in watching, and being late for their afternoon shifts. Santa, as usual was never tired of waving his right arm. He possibly spent the night with his right upper limb in a mannequin poultice to relieve the ensuing daily pain. There was no royal society available for prevention of cruelty to mannequins or any such activists on their behalf!

The children citizenry accompanied by their parents paraded the street to this annual education schedule. The children were engrossed in this consciousness experience with dripping ice cream cones in their hands and running noses. The nasal drip appeared to contribute to the flavour of the ice cream.

James and Freda decided to have a small Christmas party for James' office and hospital staff at their home in Charlestown. Freida would organise the catering to include finger foods and canapes with help from Fiona and Faye and the office girls, Shonie, Miriam and Jane. James would look after the alcoholic beverages. Among the invitees were Rowan his fellow, his registrar, Dr Mick Hall, the resident Dr. Peter Able and James' co-surgeons, Dr Eleanor McEwen with her partner, Zac and Damien White with his wife, Laura. Shonie, Miriam and Jane came with their partners.

The party music was loud and exploding with *Bing Crosby* singing, *White Christmas* followed by *Andy Williams* and *Johnny Mathis* making their contribution to incite a festive mood. It was obvious from the start that both the elder girls, Fiona and Faye had their sights set on Rowan who wore blue pants and a smart shirt and an orange silk tie, his favourite attire. The other residents were casually dressed in consideration of the hot weather.

Food and alcohol went around till some degree of inebriation was satisfactorily achieved. The one liner jokes began to flow in and some laughter echoed.

James began," Neutron walks into a bar. How much for a beer? For you, no charge."

Not to be outdone, Damien, "The past, present, and future walk into a bar. The atmosphere was tense."

Freida had one to offer, "Tennis ball walks into a bar. The bartender asks, are you being served?"

After a while, as the alcohol began to affect the prefrontal lobes, the jokes took a mild turn towards vulgarity.

Damien took his turn first, "Listen to this folks. Rob was at a fancy restaurant in London. After a few drinks, he couldn't hold back, and let out a loud long musical fart. Lord Humphrey sitting at the next table with his wife was outraged. 'How dare you fart before my wife?' Rob replied, 'My profound apologies, Sir. I did not know it was her turn next.'

Everyone laughed including Rowan.

Zac was next with his joke,

"I have one for you. The only cow in a small town in Dyess, Arkansas stopped giving milk. The people found another cow in Hazard Nebraska which they bought to replace their cow. The new cow was great and produced lots of milk, and the people were pleased and happy. They next decided to acquire a bull to mate with the cow. They bought a bull and put it in the pasture with their new cow. However whenever the bull came close to the cow, the cow would move away. No matter what approach the bull tried, the cow would move away from the bull and the bull could not succeed in his attempts. The people decided to ask the vicar, what to do. The vicar thought about this for a minute and inquired, 'Did you buy this cow in Nebraska?'

The Vet was amazed and asked 'How did you know we got the cow in Nebraska?'

The vicar replied with a distant look in his eye, 'My wife is from Nebraska.'

The laughter exploded particularly from the males. Rowan pretended he did not hear the punch line.

Rowan did restrict his alcohol intake so could remain sober in his consultant's presence.

On seeing Rowan, Fiona noticed that she felt a certain flushing, trembling and palpitations which were not emotions she had dealt with before. The girls at school sometimes talked about it but Fiona had shelfed it away as fantasy which was available in the *Mills and Bloom* books. Gaining some control of herself, Fiona approached and sat on the empty seat next to Rowan.

"Hi, I am Fiona, James' eldest daughter."

"My name is Rowan DeCruz. I am your father's fellow at the hospital. Your father is my lodestar. My father was a plastic surgeon too. He died in a plane crash."

"I am sorry to hear that. My dad always brags about how good you are at your work."

"Well, I try."

"I believe you are from India?"

"Yes, Bombay to be precise."

"What's India like? I have always wanted to see India."

"You must see it for yourself. You will like India."

"Do you practice yoga?"

"India is the birthplace of yoga but I do not practice yoga."

"Do you play cricket?"

"I did when I was in school. But not anymore."

"My grandfather, mum's father, loves to watch the Indian cricket team."

"Yes, we do have a fine team currently."

"Can you speak Hindu?"

"You mean Hindi language. Don't you? Hindu is a religious sect."

"Yes can you speak Hindi?"

"Enough to save my life and yours too if need be."

They both laughed together.

"We have about twenty three official languages including English in India."

"Wow, how do you manage to understand each other?"

"We don't," Rowan decided to be funny.

"Do you play chess?" Rowan asked.

"No."

"Chess originated in India."

"Really."

" Also Indian cuisine is the best. You will love it. 'Indian food' varies widely from place to place in the country. In Goa, from where my family hails we have a lot of Portuguese-inspired dishes."

"There are some Indian restaurants here in Newcastle. But we do not go there often. Mum is not very fond of Indian food."

"India as you possibly know is well-known for the Taj Mahal. This monument was built by Emperor Shah Jahan in memory of his wife, Mumtaz. It has the distinction of being one of the Seven Wonders of the World."

"I'd love to see the Taj Mahal one day."

"You must see it. It is fantastic. Have I given you enough reasons why you should visit?"

"If I come, will you show me around?"

"Most definitely."

"Deal?"

"Deal."

"Enough jokes. We should dance now," Freida tried to take control and pirouetted towards James. Soon they were both dancing and were joined by Damien and Laura.

Fatima was able to partner with Dr. Peter Able and really could have danced all night! Peter was a very impressive dancer and Fatima was no less at least tonight! Peter was still recovering from a severe bout of adolescence. He could pulp John Travolta into fiction with his dancing, and Fatima and he, could together release a new dance version of *Grease* provided Peter was not required to grease his retro pond hair.

Faye watched and chose to abstain from dancing and preferred to hum to the deafening music.

The music drifted to The Beatles, "*Love me do*' and "*I want to hold your hand*" and the like and the other girls also joined in with their partners. Fiona asked Rowan to dance but as expected he declined.

"I am very sorry, I don't know how to dance properly," he responded, although Rowan had been familiar with all the dance steps which he had learnt at the dancing parties in Byculla which he often attended in his adolescent years. He did not want to be seen messing with the boss' daughter for obvious reasons. The consequences could be disastrous for his career. He did not want to jeopardise that. His mother had warned him that it would break her heart if he married a foreign girl and always to have his career in mind first.

"You don't have to do anything, just shake your hands and legs a bit," Fiona was assiduous in her request.

Rowan eventually capitulated and impressed Fiona with his movements.

She noticed that his movements were similar to her own dad's.

"You dance like dad."

"I am honoured you think so."

Fiona was also fascinated by his accent. Rowan did not have a clue of Fiona's forthright effort in gaining his attention. He had been subject to such similar approaches before at the hospital and in particular, by an Italian nurse, Maria who seeking to conquer his interest, often inquired of him, "So Rowan what are you doing after work tonight?"

"I have some reading to do," was his usual honest reply.

After several such attempts, Maria shifted her attention to greener territory without Rowan even noticing the change. Maria thought Rowan may perhaps have homosexual inclinations.

James was watching the progress of Fiona's advances with Rowan and was not pleased with the possible outcome. Although he would have loved to have Rowan as his son in law, under the circumstances it would be a disaster. He must not let this relationship ripen and he was determined to end it. But how? He could not recruit Freida's aid this time. He must do it only by himself. But how?

The party progressed and both the physical and mental spirits were high all around, till very late. Eventually the guests sought leave after thanking Freida and James and showering the usual festive chants in tandem, before dissipation.

That night James could not sleep. Although the night was hot he was really bothered by Fiona's attempts for Rowan's romantic attention. Could he have predicted this? Not really. He didn't think that Fiona would be enthralled by Rowan and his unromantic methodology. He could not admonish Rowan. He knew from experience that things can be simple initially, but soon begin to spiral. He remembered his relationship with Carmen. He was responsible for making her life miserable. Nevertheless Rowan was her reward and she had done very well, I admire you Carmen, he thought.

But now he had to deal with Fiona and the current problem. But how? He decided he would deal with Fiona at breakfast in front of the whole family.

Rowan also had a problem with going to sleep. However his problem was of a very different kind. He had promised Fiona that he would look after her if she came to India for a visit. He now wished he had not enumerated to her the advantages of seeing India. He blamed the alcohol which he was sure he had tried to curtail. What if she really took up his offer after he left Australia and arrived in Byculla? This would be a problem for him. What would his mother say? What would his uncle Cecil and Esther say? Had he put his foot in? How was he going to get out without causing damage to his own career and with her father, James? Hopefully he would never see her again. Such thoughts bothered him until sleep eventually took over.

Faye was also having her own problems going off to sleep and the heat of the night was not conducive. She had noted Rowan was cute and Fiona had dominated his attention for all of the evening. She had not even managed to say hello to him. Should she have made her presence known? Should she have had a cat fight with Fiona over Rowan? Why is the eldest always the most advantaged? What should she do? She had always loved and respected Fiona. And so Fiona gets him, she decided. Even if she has to join the holy order of spinsterhood in this particular matter.

Fatima and Freida were both very tired and had no issues to contend with and drifted off to sleep with no effort at all.

Breakfast was late at the Regan household the next morning with the usual attendees being summoned by repeated reminders by Freida. James was sitting at the table when Fiona arrived.

"Hi everyone" Fiona introduced herself apparently quite pleased with last night's outcome.

"Fiona I need to talk you about Rowan."

"Rowan, your fellow? Gee dad, he is trying so hard to be like you. He even rolls his tongue just like you. His movements are just like you. I like him"

"I would prefer you not to have any romantic involvement with him. It makes my work with him very much harder."

"Really? How?"

"Imagine if you came and worked with me."

"Heaven forbid. Hell no. But the analogy does not hold here dad."

"He will be subject to nepotism complaints from the others. He is very good at his work and that will weigh on his talent."

Fiona felt crestfallen but she could understand what her father was hinting at. Yes, that would not help

Rowan in his career. She had to succumb to the advice as she would be impeding Rowan's progress.

Freida was looking hard at James, as she would also have loved to have Rowan as her eldest son in law. She would discuss this later with James in close quarters. There must be a way out here to welcome Rowan into our family, she thought.

Later in very close quarters, Freida inquired, "Why do you not approve of Rowan for Fiona?"

"I thought I had made myself clear. It would not be fair to Rowan. He has made a lot of sacrifices to be here. He has given up time with his family to be here to advance his career possibilities when he gets back home to India. We can't drag him astray."

Freida could see what James was hinting at.

"Sorry, I was just being selfish," Freida concluded and rolled off to sleep.

When Rowan saw James at the hospital next time, "Thank you very much for inviting me to your Christmas party sir. I enjoyed it very much."

"I am glad you enjoyed it Rowan and thank you for coming. I am a bit busy right now. I must run. I will see you later."

"That's fine sir."

The boss thanked me for coming to his party, Rowan thought. This would never happen in India. I am so lucky. Maybe grandma is looking after me from heaven. He turned his eyes towards heaven. Thank you grandma. And he remembered the times he had with his grandma in Byculla and how she had always advised him wisely. A tear came to his eyes.

Rowan like most Indians was also addicted to conspiracy theories or rather conspiracy fallacies or fantasies. He thought his dead grandma had conspired with his dead dad to make his life lucky. He also knew this conspiration may not have happened if she was still alive today. Some things have to happen for other things to happen. He particularly remembered how she often rosaried to him, 'If you don't take advantage of your advantages, you will lose them'. Just now how he hoped for some of his own luck to rub onto his own mother! I wish she was here with me!

He must write to his mum tonight and tell her about the boss' Christmas party.

23

It was decided that Fatima would go to boarding school in Sydney for her final two years of high school. This would provide her with the best chance of securing the requisite scores for medical school admission. She obtained admission and started as a boarder at a school in Wahroonga. After the initial new school hiccups, she soon settled.

She loved the school and participated in whatever activities she could find time for including studying English, higher mathematics, physics, chemistry and geology. She enjoyed the 'rocks in the head' feeling with geology.

The schedules allowed the girls to go home on the weekends to allow the school cooks enough time to revise their allegiance to the least appetising recipe manifestos.

That Sunday, Freida had just dropped Fatima off at the school gate, she, having spent the weekend at home in Charlestown. Freida was driving back on her way home now. She was stationary at the traffic lights at Hornsby waiting to get on to the highway to Newcastle.

Suddenly she was hit in the rear by another vehicle.

She heard a loud bang and felt a forward thrust movement to her neck during the hit, causing her forehead to collide with the steering wheel. She felt momentarily dazed and a massive headache ensued immediately.

She drove her car on to the shoulder lane and parked. She got out and examined the damage to the car. She was surprised that there was almost none. The other woman driver appeared to be in her late adolescence. She parked her Toyota just behind Freida and came towards her with an apologetic face, "I am very sorry."

"That's okay. There does not seem to be much damage on my car. Nevertheless I will have it checked at the garage tomorrow." She brought a notebook out of her pocket. "I need your phone number and I will note your car registration. I don't think we will call the police."

"Okay. Here's my telephone and I am insured with GIO," the other driver wrote her number in Freida's notebook.

"I will ring you," Freida closed, attempting to ignore the headache. Both then drove away from the site.

On the way back, the headache persisted and she was also feeling nauseous now. Should she stop and call James? It was Sunday. He should be home. No, she could manage till she got home. Why bother him and cause him to worry? No, she will drive home and put with this bloody massive headache till then.

She got home and explained it all to James.

"Stupid kids," he irated, "They let them out on the road before they can hardly read the colours of the traffic signals."

He brought her some Panadol tablets which she swallowed with some water expecting relief. But the headache was relentless with its new capture and refused to be tamed.

Further medication provided was of no avail. She rested all day in the bedroom with a minimal appetite and a sleepless night ensued.

She saw her local medical practitioner in the morning who advised imaging studies of the head and neck which showed no significant abnormality. She was prescribed further stronger pain medication and requested to return back in a couple of days.

With no relief in sight, on next day after another sleepless night, James rang the neurosurgeon, Dr. Peter Rosenberg at his rooms and asked if he could bring in his wife too see him that morning.

"Of course, James. Can you come at eleven?"

"I shall be there with her."

Peter Rosenberg examined her and looked at the radiographs.

"The radiographs do not show any bone fracture or displacement. I think the problem is facet joint injury which usually does not show on films."

"Then what will reduce this headache at the back of my neck which does not allow me to rest or sleep?" Freida inquired.

"I think I will give you some stronger pain killers

and you can use some heat application. Hopefully that will work."

The heat provided some temporary relief initially but this faded in time.

Freida had difficulty sleeping and when she did fall asleep she woke up in abject pain. She felt miserable all day. James also noticed she was getting emotionally numb towards him. She requested him to move into another bedroom. She felt his snoring was not helping. He was struggling to understand her, his beloved Freida, was slowly drifting away from him. She was very taciturn and very irritable and very temperamental. She always felt tired and washed out. She preferred to be left alone. A persistent headache and lack of sleep did not allow her to contribute to her household obligations either. The older girls who were at home sympathised and helped as much as possible but their efforts were importunately faulted with acerbic remarks from Freida. The girls usually ran for cover and went out or locked themselves in their rooms to escape her unpredictable moods. James was not spared. He adapted by waking up early and left early to grab a coffee and doughnuts at the shops on the way to work. He returned home late.

Over two months Freida worsened and was falling into a deep depression. Her general practitioner diagnosed post-traumatic stress disorder and prescribed Tofranil. The medication did not seem to affect her irritability. She spent long hours in bed now and began nursing suicidal thoughts. But how? The method would have to be by mouth. She was not brave enough to be able to inject herself. She thought about the junkies. How did they manage it? She only had access to Tofranil. What about Tofranil and alcohol? Alcohol in larger doses with any mind altering drug is usually toxic. Maybe I could try that. Then for a moment she would ponder. These are stupid thoughts. I must rid myself of them. I want to be there for Fiona's, Faye's and Fatima's weddings. I want to see my grandchildren. But I can't live with this pain. There is no end to this pain. New thoughts flowed.

James was in the theatre dressing room with Rowan when he was paged.

"Doctor Regan can you ring switch immediately," the voiced echoed.

James was irritated. Who could want him now?

He moved toward the telephone and dialled switch.

"We have a call for you doctor. I'm putting it through."

"Yes"

"Dad can you come home soon, mum is not well."

"Faye, what is the matter?"

"It's mum. It was very quiet. So I checked in the bedroom. She is not breathing."

"Call the ambulance. I am coming home right away," and he hung up.

"Rowan you will have to manage this afternoon. There is an emergency at home. I have to go."

Rowan had barely got to his feet to acknowledge when James raced out in his theatre clothes to his car.

When he arrived home Freida was already pronounced dead by the ambulance.

James' heart sank. His Freida was no more. This

was Freida who had said 'life is for living'. His beloved Freida. Why did she leave him? Could he join her? How will he manage without her?

Tears welled heavily in his eyes. Was he responsible? For not heeding her pain? For avoiding her? Should he have stayed at home to look after her? If he had done that, maybe then this would not have happened. What now? I have the girls and... and I have Rowan when I tell him.

Regarding the funeral arrangements, there was a mild disagreement with Grace who wanted Freida to be buried in catholic soil. However James felt Freida would not have liked that and he was not going to let her down now. Fred, whose religious affiliations were usually dictated by Grace, abstained from the argument, either oblivious or unconcerned of the later consequences to him of this decision, from Grace's wrath.

Following the funeral James took some time off from work. The days and particularly the nights at home were hard. Often in bed at night, he would roll over and expect to find Freida. She's just gone to the toilet he would think and will be back soon. At times he felt bitterness towards Freida for leaving him. There was no logic in his thinking. If I had cared for her more, this would not have happened. If only I had not gone to work on that day, this would not have happened. Rowan could have managed at work. It is entirely all my fault.

In the mornings he felt foggy, heavy and confused.

What am I without Freida? Nothing. She was the pillar that I leaned on. I am so lucky that I had so many beautiful years with her. She will always live in my memories. Maybe I should go back to work. That may help me to cope with life a bit better.

Downhearted and depressed he managed to push himself back at work. Everyday life became more of the same. Rowan understood his plight and took over as much as he could to help.

Fatima went back to boarding school and was very determined to keep her promise to her demised mum. To this end her books prevailed over her other commitments and her teachers noticed the change and were very pleased with her dedication.

However back at home for the holidays, Fatima suddenly decided she did not want to go back to boarding school and wanted to stay at home in Charlestown to be with the rest of the family. No amount of coaxing from the other members of the family would make her change her mind.

She was able to gain admission at a local school. Fatima was dux of the school in Year eleven which brought some joy into James' life. I wish Freida was here, he thought.

Fatima's studious habits persisted and she was dux again in Year twelve. She did extremely well at the Higher School Certificate Exam and got admission into medical school at Sydney University but decided to take a gap year off from study.

Meanwhile James slowly managed to put some order into his inchoate life. He resorted to reading philosophy which he hoped would reinvigorate him and occupy his thinking. He started with *Immanuel Kant* and noted that Kant argued that there were only two ways of knowing, one by way of our senses and the other, by reasoning. He noted that Kant described the world as we experience it, as phenomenal and the world as it actually is, as noumenal. The former requires concepts of time, space and causality. It is not possible for us to know the noumenal world as it lacks things in particular or is undifferentiated. James thought that perhaps 'near death experiences' are visits to the noumenal world?

Next he chose to read *Arthur Schopenhauer*. Basically he found that Schopenhauer is an escapist and attempts to provide an escape from reality by four methods, *Aesthetic contemplation*, the effectiveness of which is of a fixed time. Next the *cultivation of sympathy* by recognising that we as humans are all the victims of the same relentless suffering. In this case also the effectiveness is temporary. The next technique Schopenhauer recommends is *music*, with which James totally agreed and *finally the need to lose the 'Will to live'* which he felt was a bit harsh. This was the option Freida chose which hurt him most of all. He concluded that Schopenhauer's philosophies are really confessions of the philosopher's own temperament and are not really objective insights into valid life strategies. Except for the music perhaps.

Next he turned his attention to *Søren Kierkegaard*.

Whilst previous philosophers thought of man belonging to something larger than oneself, Kierkegaard put the focus back on the individual. Kierkegaard was himself a fervently religious man. He claimed that the fundamental problem everyone must first face is boredom. A wholehearted, single-minded, and undistracted commitment to God, a leap of faith, was Kierkegaard's conception of the only complete life. Been there, done that, James thought. Kierkegaard claimed that we reach a certain point where we may find that, who we are keeps us from becoming who we are. Kierkegaard also said that there are no moral phenomena, only moral interpretations of phenomena. James could agree with that.

He was also impressed by *Martin Heidegger* who maintained that only through a true comprehension of our finitude with eventual death, can we find our authenticity which involves discovering what are truly one's own unique life possibilities. Hence an inauthentic existence involves a fleeing from what are one's own individual possibilities. Inauthentic existence involves living amidst the routine and the conventional. James found this concept interesting.

James had deciphered that philosophy bore a complex relationship to religion, especially in its institutionalized forms. He had worked out that these early philosophers were mainly influenced by their Christian upbringing and not really relevant in today's world. Perhaps such philosophy had reached an ersatz status in our current times! Advances in the sciences made more and more domains amenable to empirical investigation, which raised the questions as to whether the subject matter of philosophy should exist anymore. The questions to which philosophy provided answers in the past were now redundant, lost, muted, or superseded. Even some aspects of religion in its traditional forms spoke to concerns that we no longer have, have outgrown, or have lost touch with. We have moved from issues regarding death through to concerns regarding guilt, to an era in which the presence or absence of meaning in human life has become central, James thought. Also biotechnological opportunities, passing out from the status of science fiction to that of actual possibility, have raised major questions regarding what it actually means to be human. Interesting food for thought he thought!

One night as he was lying in bed, a thought rolled in his head. May be there is an opportunity for him to invite Rowan into his family. He had gone quite fond of Rowan and eventually Rowan was his own and only son. He could not let him go back and get lost in the Indian shenaniganry. He would go to Bombay now and find Carmen and suggest to her to marry him and come with him to Australia. She may never agree, which is the most likely outcome, after the way he had treated her. She would be crazy to ever him trust again. But then, it may work. He remembered her as quite attractive then and maybe hopefully now too! Nothing could be lost in trying. He remembered their good times in Bombay. Perhaps it would work! He had only hope on his side.

Rowan had informed James in one of their

conversations that his mother had obtained a degree in Psychology and done brilliantly at it. James remembered Carmen's thinking was always of a high calibre in all the argumentation that they had embarked upon, in those days. Perhaps he should read some Freudian theory to aid his efforts and establish a mutual conversational topicality, in case she concurs to associate with him. Although he had vaguely explored Freud before he set himself the task of analysing Freudian theory further. He was now able to see how Freud construes human life as the relentless disappointment of deep human needs. Freud also identified some deeply hidden human instincts such as the incestuous, the cannibalistic, and the homicidal. Overall he found Sigmund Freud interesting including his work on dreams. He was also aware that most of Freud's work on psychoanalysis and dreams was no longer accepted by experts for want of scientific evidence. However he still admired Freud's method of thinking in his time. He loved *Professor John Kihlstrom's* quote on Freud, '*More than Einstein or Watson and Crick, more than Hitler or Lenin, Roosevelt or Kennedy, more than Picasso, Eliot, or Stravinsky, more than the Beatles or Bob Dylan, Freud's influence on modern culture has been profound and long-lasting.*' He himself was not in a position to comment on this matter yet!

Having done the mandatory homework, James planned to take two weeks off and go to India to meet Carmen. Depending on the situational circumstances, he would inveigle her into marrying him. As per the astrology "moon" character he was, conferred on him by Janet his sister, no one was advised about his schedule, except that he was going to go away for a holiday and would be back at work in two weeks time. If it works, he may have a wife again!

24

James arrived at Santa Cruz Airport amid the usual locally manufactured chaos. He tried hard to be oblivious of all the sights and sounds around. But India being what it is, is very intrusive into all the human senses and any defences are worthless. Soon his auditory senses were inundated by the Indian music at the airport which easily exceeded the safe decibel levels. The mixed smells of the Indian spices and the human sweat wafted through, challenging any olfactory blocks. Even the visual sensation was not spared by the multi-coloured sequined saris and their occupants. Give up, the atmosphere implored of him! Admit it you have lost!

Having cleared the official entry impediments, James thoughts attempted to take a different direction. Does Carmen's family surname have anything to do with Santa Cruz airport? Maybe they had a saint in the family? But no, that can wait.

Other pressing matters needed attention first. Just outside the airport, the smells of urine, cow dung, spices, sandalwood incense fought for recognition in his nose and the incessant car horns with no other intention but only to deter silence, claimed possession of his hearing. He was in now in spiritual India, a whole nation and people devoid of reality, a notion that he had once worked out in his initial encounters.

Amid the expected taxi and road chaos he finally found his accommodation at The Taj Hotel at Colaba. Back in the room he unpacked and adorned himself for the task at hand. He was in a hurry to see Carmen and decided to take a taxi to Byculla.

"I don't think I ever want to see you again. Just leave me alone," Carmen roared at him.

"I want you to know something," James begged.

"You have no right to talk to me ever again after what you put me through," Carmen shouted at him.

"You are right but I need to tell you something."

"You left me with a pregnancy and didn't bother to find out what happened to me or the child. You didn't have the guts to deal with the problems that you created. You were not man enough to face my family. You just disappeared without trace. And now you have come back after all these years. Do you even know you have a son who is a plastic surgeon and is now studying in Australia?" she said loudly.

"I very much want to apologise and explain. I have been sorry every day of my life, Carmen. Please, I need to tell you about our son, Rowan who is studying in my department in Australia?"

At the mention of Rowan's name Carmen's mood changed entirely. She was pleased that Rowan had met his untrustworthy father and at the same time she did not want to upset Rowan's boss and jeopardise Rowan's future. She felt that she did not know enough of this man to risk that.

"I need to explain. Can we meet tomorrow at six at

Kit Kat restaurant?"

"I need to think about that. No more hanky panky from you this time."

"No more hanky panky, I promise. Can we meet?"

She took some time to decide, "Okay I will see you there."

This time again James arrived early.

"Hello Carmen."

Carmen abhorred his friendliness. She will not let her emotions go astray this time after all the mental trauma she had been through in her last encounter with this man. She had learned never to trust any man except her brother and Rowan. It was only for Rowan's sake she was here.

She remembered the time when the local Romeos used to chant when she passed by in her pregnant state, "Here comes the Blessed Virgin Carmen. Let us pray for her." How angry she had felt at that time. She could physically decapitate each one of them and make them bleed to kosher or halal. How could this person with her today have been so inhuman?

"Hi," she replied

They went in and were escorted to a table. The waiter somehow sensed the prevailing atmosphere and left quickly, "I come back when you ready."

"I can appreciate why you are so angry with me and rightly so," James began.

"How is Rowan?"

"Rowan is good. A very good lad. He is my fellow and works with me. I keep a very close eye on him. He is the finest person I know. Thanks entirely to you

Carmen."

"I am grateful to my mother for that. From the time he was born and till he went to medical school she took complete control of him. She went back to work just to educate Rowan. God bless her."

"I wish I had met her."

"You bastard."

After Cecil's warning, she knew he employed his charm and politeness as evasive qualities that concealed the truth about him.

James on his part realised he was in enemy territory. This would be a very difficult mission. He had never been in such a situation before.

"Would you like to visit Rowan in Australia? I can make the arrangements for you to do that if you wish?"

She thought, can I ever trust this bastard again?

"I need to think about it."

"Of course."

Noticing the mood was changing the waiter reappeared and inquired if choices had been made.

"Give us another minute," James responded.

They made their choices promptly and the waiter was summoned and took their order.

Carmen was taciturn and in a pensive mood. What if I go and he dumps me again, there? Rowan was there already and he would help me. But what if James has poisoned Rowan's mind? Not Rowan, nobody could poison Rowan against his family. We are a family first. This bastard tried to stuff my family for me, several years ago but never again will I allow him to do that.

The food arrived and was devoured at a very fast pace. James settled the bill.

"Can I pay my share?" Carmen inquired.

"No Carmen, it was my idea."

On the way out James queried, "When will you let me know?"

"Tomorrow. I need time to think."

"Do you want to meet me here again or do you want to come to the Taj Hotel?"

Carmen would very much have liked to go to the Taj Hotel but her better self said, no. It was too close to his abode and if she did have an alcoholic drink with him then he was capable of taking advantage of her again. Like he did before. Just not worth the risk.

"Here at six. Bye."

"Yeah. Bye."

On the way back she was thrilled with the idea of going to Australia and meeting her darling, Rowan. She had already made up her mind.

The meal next day was merely to confirm her assent. With James sitting across her, her heart was beginning to recondition. Could she fall in love with James again? Never, she reaffirmed to herself. No way. But then I wonder how his life is going on now? She wanted to know.

"So how is your practice going on in Australia?"

"Very good."

"Are you married now?"

"I was. My wife is dead."

"I am sorry to hear that. Have you any children?"

"I have three daughters, Fiona, Faye and Fatima . And our son Rowan."

Carmen was not sure she heard correctly. She saw a propitiousity in his mention of Rowan. She was not sure. She was heavily scorched once and could not afford to go for a second helping.

"Are you planning to marry again?"

"Only if you will accept?"

Carmen was not sure that she heard correctly. Nevertheless she wanted to make no more mistakes.

"I'm sorry, I don't want to see those days again, never, ever again. I am sure about that."

"Have you decided about visiting Rowan?"

"Yes, I will accept that offer from you but with absolutely no strings attached."

Later that evening back at the hotel, James decided to visit the bar. He found the décor in the bar was most fascinating and appealing. He could just sit and stare at it.

He ordered a double Johnny Walker whiskey on the rocks and was just beginning to help it find its way within him when he was intercepted by an American accented voice, "Hello sir, my name is Omar. May I join you?"

James did not recognise the bearded owner of the face on which only a prominent nose demanded all of the attention. The man was holding a drink, which had a junipery scent and was perhaps a gin. James would have preferred to deal with his lugubriousity alone but under the circumstances soon recognised he had no choice.

"Sure, take a seat. My name is James."

"My name is Omar. I am from Lahore in Pakistan. I am here for a meeting of Gevaert Film executives."

James had seen the Welcome to Gevaert employees posters in the lobby but had not given it a second thought. He had not even heard of Gevaert before. He decided that was not going to be interested now.

"I am a plastic surgeon from Australia," James continued.

"Perhaps this is a stupid question but what brings you to India?"

James was not prepared, "I'm just passing through. I note you have an American accent."

"Yes, I was in Wisconsin for six long years. I did a major on Samuel Clemens *aka* Mark Twain and as if that is not enough, my wife is an American and also has a major in Mark Twain."

"And you twain shall meet," James added his own brand of humour with a small laugh to reinforce.

Omar liked the little joke and contributed with a complimentary smile, "Have you read Mark Twain?"

"I have read *Innocents Abroad* and enjoyed his humour. And who has not read *Tom Sawyer* and *Adventures of Huckleberry Finn*?"

"*Innocents Abroad* was the best-selling of all his books during his lifetime."

"Really," James was surprised.

"Mark Twain was essentially a travel writer. He knew that travel writing could present all kinds of opportunities for laughter by creating all kinds of misunderstandings and misadventures, from trying to communicate in another language to trying to enjoy an especially exotic foreign cuisine."

"Oh yes I can see that now," James agreed.

"Twain tends to dramatise the misunderstanding between a set of preconceptions and a series of new circumstances of travel, or between the ideas of the world a traveller has in his mind before and the unfamiliar realities he meets on the journey. And as he himself admits, 'Travel is fatal to prejudice' and uses this to create his humour. He thus felt laughter could serve as a way to destroy falsehoods and liberate the mind."

"That is so true for westerners when they see the east."

"Unfortunately Twain was most interested in becoming rich and that affected his later writing. His imagination was continuously obliged to think in terms of popularity, salability, and audience expectations. Decisions about what to write, or what to delete from or leave in his texts, were often business decisions rather than artistic ones."

"Authors like Henry James wrote cautionary tales of American innocence and optimism challenged by the complexity and suffering of human experience," James opined.

"In fact Mark Twain sets out to liberate his readers from impressions imposed by Henry James and others. He attacks these books in a variety of moods from burlesque to parody to irony to satire and even polemic."

"Indeed," James responded.

"If you have noted he presents his critique of the Bible particularly, very carefully, anxious not to shock the audience he was trying to entertain as well as instruct. His views are summarised for example when he says, 'imagination labours best in distant fields.' Also you say you have read *Huck Finn*. What did you think about it?"

"I read it a long time ago. I loved it. But after listening to you Omar, I am too afraid to venture an opinion on Twain. In fact I am looking forward to your critique," James said.

"To me considering that the novel was written after slavery was effectively abolished, it is almost a treatise on anti-racism."

"I'm sorry you will have to explain that to me in a bit more detail," James said.

"Well, the popular opinion is that Twain wrote Huck Finn to liberate American literature from British conventions. The language is authentic derived from his own experience. And in the first person narration you can't get any closer to the truth."

"I like it when, instead of deferring to books as "authorities," Huck tests their claims against his own experience. For example, when he experiments to see if both prayer and rubbing a lamp will work," James continued.

"Twain is as much interested in the fictions of Huck's culture as in the derived fictions it conveys. For example the cultural belief that slavery is right and approved by god. It is because Huck starts largely outside the "regular" conventions of society, and relies chiefly on his own experience, that he is able to see Jim more clearly. Initially believing that values from god and society demanded that Jim be treated as property that can be bought and sold from, he realises on the raft trip that Jim is a very much a human being like him. When Huck plays that trick on him, the conversation that plays relays friendship, equality, and human dignity and essentially reality. Can you see how the antiracism card is being played here?"

"As I see it now, both Jim and Huck have problems. Jim's problem is physical in escaping slavery; Huck's problem is mental in escaping societal values," James added.

"That's exactly it. Huck sees slavery in the way his society does, as being right, and approved by god and conditioned by his society's prejudices. Even his self-image is the one he had been given by his society," Omar continued.

"Yes there is a significant conflict between what Huck has been taught or trained to think and what he learns from his own experience and feelings," James remarked.

"When Huck decides to "go to hell" to help Jim to freedom" is perhaps the high point of the novel," Omar finished.

"I know now what you mean by antiracist notes in the novel."

The conversation had occupied them both and they both realised that they had not found time to finish their drinks.

Big gulps, in attempts to empty the glasses followed.

"I found that very interesting Omar. I am so glad I met you. Perhaps you can tell me a bit more about yourself. Do you live in Lahore now?"

"No we live between Lahore and Richmond, Virginia in the US. My wife and I met as freshmen. We have a daughter. She is now one year old."

"I have three daughters"

Omar provided a look of sympathy towards James. James thought that maybe because, Omar himself was also still locked in his own societal values.

"We thought we would settle in Pakistan. But my wife just does not like it there."

"Why?" James inquired.

"The perpetual corruption, cheating and crime that begins with the politicians down to the common man, gets her. There does not seem to be any hope or a way out for both Pakistan and India. The Indian politicians have a unique way of lying to the uneducated populace and telling them India is the best country in the world. According to them, India discovered everything a long time ago. It is all given in the *Vedas*. In Pakistan the usual method is by eliminating the dissenters."

The conversation now was beginning to follow the usual route in regard to these two countries. He had heard it all before amongst the surgical residents in Leeds. Maybe he should excuse himself now.

"Well, Omar I must go. It was very nice meeting you and I learned a lot from you today."

"My pleasure. Goodbye, enjoy you trip."

They shook hands and James took the lift to his room on the sixth floor from where he ordered the dinner room service, as he wished to have a solitary meal and could not risk having any more company in the restaurants below.

After the meal, as he lay in bed, he thought about Omar and *Huck Finn*. That was an informative conversation he thought before drifting off to sleep.

Carmen's travel visa was applied for and tickets arranged for by James before he left for Sydney. There may be a chance he thought. She may change her mind. The probability exists. It was arranged that she will stay in an apartment with Rowan in Newcastle.

After James left, Carmen went off to see Cecil and discuss the matter with him. Cecil although apprehensive at first, soon fell in with the idea and even proposed that if Carmen was still attracted to him then she should consider marrying James.

"No Cecil, after what I have been through that is most unlikely"

Cecil understood.

25

James was back in Australia and at work. He informed Rowan that he had visited his mother during a recent trip to India and met his mother and had invited her to visit him here in Australia and that she had accepted. Rowan could not believe his ears. To accommodate Carmen on her arrival, Rowan was relocated to an apartment in Mayfield by James. Rowan was delighted with the new place which had a lounge, two bedrooms and a kitchen and an allocated parking spot. Rowan could not contain his joy and thanked James profusely.

"You are so kind sir," Rowan rolled his tongue.

"Just trying," James replied rolling his tongue.

At this moment he just wanted to hold Rowan and give him a tight hug. He only hoped that Carmen will forgive him and accept his offer of marriage but was imminently reminded of her last, 'never ever' words. Little hope. But if she consented all his problems would be over and hers too, he thought.

Carmen arrived in Sydney and was porschcd to Mayfield by James after she cleared all the passport and customs formalities at the airport. She had carried with her some of the spice ingredients from India for Rowan's favourite curries and managed to get them through the custom enforcement authorities. She was quite pleased with her success, as she was warned by Cecil of the very strict Australian Customs.

Carmen was awed by the relative absence of noise as she walked out. She invited her olfaction to participate in the perfumed smells of the passing travellers. Her eyeballs pleaded to be let out of their restraining sockets to absorb in all the available cues including the advertisements for, '*I still call Australia home*' at the airport terminal.

James was pleased to see her and implanted a bold kiss on her lips to which she did not object. The presence of the people around may have prompted her reaction. She was in a different country. In Rome do as the Romans do, she thought.

On his part, there is hope, he thought.

On the way back, their conversation was restricted to comparing India with Australia. James hoped to opinionate Carmen into Australia's favour for obvious reasons.

"India is constipated with people and the only laxative that works is corruption and bribery," James said.

"That's our system of governance," Carmen agreed laughingly.

He played Crosby, Stills, Nash and Young, *Teach Your Children*, hoping to cause a tear at her heart.

She listened to the music but did not comment. She had not heard the song before.

They finally arrived at the rented apartment at

Mayfield and James unlocked and showed her in. He had equipped it very basically for Rowan and her, hoping they would move in with him soon. So far he had no indication from Carmen that his plan was working. But then, it was still too early.

James remembered that there was a *hare jesus* variety place of worship in the vicinity at the Mayfied apartment that may attract Carmen. He decided to let her find it out for herself if she felt the need to. He left her alone in the apartment after providing some basic domestic instructions.

Rowan met his mother later that evening after work. Both mother and son soon indulged in an endless conversation reminiscing about their Byculla days.

"This is a nice country mum. Everyone is very good to me, specially Dr Regan," Rowan opened.

"For a reason Rowan."

"What do you mean?"

"He is your father," Carmen replied.

"What?"

Rowan was shocked and looked into her eyes. He felt a multitude of emotions assaulting him at the same moment. Unbelievable. How can it be? He was looking for a further clue in his mother's face. This was too much for him to take in. Although he felt a sudden internal satisfaction he also felt an immense anger at the same time. His father was still alive and he had met him! How lucky he was, finally. Why had his mother and grandmother never told him anything about this before! Things now began to fall into place, slowly and surely. That answered why everyone accused him of imitating James too much, in spite of his frustrating attempts not to do so. It explained why James was always on the lookout for him. Why James clandestinely cared about him. But why did James desert his mother? Was there something wrong with his mother that he himself did not know?

Several queries begged for his attention at the same time. He could not ask his mother her most intimate questions. He needed time. Anyway his beloved mother was with him now. And that was the most important thing. He wished his grandmother was here too. He ironed out that the role of his mother and grandmother in those days had been to help him cope, but not necessarily to tell him the truth. He understood. Nevertheless tonight would be sleepless he fathomed and for a long time in bed, it was. He tried hard to work out the plausible and the possible, until the waiting sleep finally took control.

Next morning before he went off to the hospital he asked Carmen if they could both go out to dinner into town that night. Carmen understood what was coming. Sooner or later she would have to face the exact truth with Rowan. Rowan was an adult and also a doctor. This would make it much easier to explain to him about her earlier sexual encounters with James. She only hoped that in narrating to Rowan, her own feelings for James would not be re-aroused. Hopefully Rowan would understand the predicament of their situation in those times, in Byculla. She did not want Rowan to have any ill feelings against

James at this stage. So she would have to modify her story a bit and exclude any blame on James. A fact when narrated to suit a point of view is essentially fiction, a fairy tale and a fairy tale it shall be.

While Rowan was at work, Carmen strolled around the suburb delighting all her senses with all the space and the relative cleanliness and the lack of noise. She was marvelled with the car yards and the multitude of cars parked within. In India these cars would have disappeared overnight, by means, fair or foul, more likely foul! She was pleased to find a catholic church in the vicinity. She was reminded of Dorothy in the *Wizard of Oz*. She went in and offered her ineluctable gratitude.

A desolate priest who was possibly on a self-guilt ablation duty approached her with a rosary in hand, "Hello. Are you visiting?"

"Yes father. I have come from India for a short stay with my son."

"What does your son do?"

"He is a plastic surgeon at the hospital."

"Which hospital?"

"Royal Newcastle Hospital."

"Does he come to our church?"

"I don't know. He has only recently moved here."

"I am expecting both of you at mass this Sunday."

"Yes father," Carmen responded and was pleased to have made a clergical acquaintance in this country.

Carmen paid her prayer dues and left the church concluding with the sign of the cross, watered down with the holy water available from the stoup. Once outside, she set her mind to the task of planning the story for Rowan tonight while multitasking her senses to the demanding surroundings.

The bus stop was barely decipherable. She realised it was a stop because a bus did stop there. For the delay, the elderly lady took in alighting and making the bus wait, it was possible that the lady owned, or was a very near relation of hers owned the bus company. The buses in Bombay usually do not allow the passengers that much time to alight. The disabled and elderly in Bombay usually avoided the buses for fear of both verbal and physical injury. She wondered if she should take a bus ride herself, just for the experience. But where would she go, apart from getting lost and causing panic and distressing Rowan. She would ask Rowan for some bus details tonight for her future use.

Further down the road she saw a poster for a *Warren Beatty* film, *Shampoo*. She had heard he was *Shirley MacLaine*'s brother. She had loved Shirley in *What a Way to Go* with *Paul Newman*. She had a closer look at Warren Beatty on the poster and decided to watch the movie with Rowan sometime before she got back to Bombay.

When she got home she wrote a letter to Cecil expressing her delight with the apartment in Mayfield, with the country and with Rowan. She also mentioned that she may watch *Warren Beatty*'s film, *Shampoo*. There was no mention of James in the letter. She had located a post office on her morning walk and decided she would walk back and post her letter.

One the way, she saw a rather obese woman who had lost most neurological control of her own anatomical connections possibly from prolonged disuse. The woman was attempting to control a quasi-pregnant obese dog. The dog was not in agreement with the route to be taken on this occasion. The chain lead bore the brunt of their disagreement and was threatening an altruistic self-immolation to settle the dispute. It is also possible that the dispute may have been related to the dog's quest for freedom and perhaps the dog wished some activists to intervene. In exchange the dog would happily part with its own chain to aid the activists' needs for chaining to trees or the like, if any.

On the way back home Carmen brought herself some cinnamon spiced doughnuts which she would enjoy with some tea.

After adequate inquiries at the hospital from colleagues, Rowan booked a table for two at a posh restaurant in town for the evening. He was determined to make this a memorable event for his mother.

When he went home that evening, Carmen was already dressed and waiting. She looked beautiful in her pink blouse and red sari. Rowan complimented her on her dress and got himself ready.

They drove to the restaurant in his Morris 850, which was the source of an inexhaustible supply of petrol smelling farts when driving. The car often reminded him of Sudhir, his medical school classmate and the car which Sudhir often drove to the JJ Hospital campus. Both cars appeared to have similar genetic attributes. After parking the car, Carmen and Rowan went into an Italian restaurant with soft music adulterating the air waves around. They were guided to the reserved table with a view of the harbour by the waiter who preferred to hide his upper lip with a black moustache just leaving enough space to make his language decipherable to non-Italians.

Rowan ordered some chilled rosé wine. The waiter left conveying the wine order to several other employees he met along the way, in the manner of a loud trade secret.

Australian cuisine was available on the menu. Rowan felt a helping of roast lamb or something similar would not challenge her taste buds adequately at this stage, although Carmen expressed a desire to try. He remembered his own early experiences in Australia when his own choices were very limited for monetary reasons.

"No mum, not this time. I want you to enjoy today. Maybe you should go for some Italian on the menu tonight."

"Okay then, you choose. I trust you."

"When we go out next time you can try Australian. Australian cuisine is catered for hunger, not enjoyment. I just want you to enjoy today. May be you should try some lasagne. I will have some too, just to prove it is safe."

"I don't want anything with noodles. I couldn't

handle it with a sari"

"No, no spaghetti."

The waiter reappeared with the wine and glasses. He placed the wine in the ice bucket and inquired about the food choices which were promptly conveyed. The waiter took some notes and left satisfied at his own scripting efforts.

Rowan filled the glasses and the usual round of "cheers" was indulged in. He was looking forward to hearing Carmen's version of 'Romeo and Juliet'. It is always interesting to hear about one's own parents' romance, just perhaps to be able to advise them how they could have done things better. Carmen had decided to introduce a fairy-tale genre to her story which suited the occasion well, as if she was reading to Rowan, when he was baby.

"Once upon a time there was a doctor called James Regan who came on a mission visit to JJ Hospital where a nurse called Carmen worked. They were both attracted to each other at first sight. He was not a frog. And she had no glass slippers and things happened as in a 'girl meets boy' story."

"And the rest is history or rather my story?" Rowan said. And Carmen immediately understood that she and James were vindicated by Rowan. Rowan did not push his queries further.

"Correct." Carmen replied. It is amazing how many lies are required to protect one truth, she thought.

"It must have been hard for you and particularly for grandma and Cecil in our grand Byculla."

"Grandma was a great woman. As you know she

lived just for you."

Rowan felt tears appear in his eyes, "You know what I mean. Grandma was the greatest woman in spite of all her rottweiler obsessions."

"Let bygones be bygones." Carmen said.

But Rowan was ready with, "And you'll fall in love once again?"

Carmen realised she had put her foot in it!

The food arrived and the waiter bon appétited them and left.

Both of them enjoyed the food. Carmen thanked Rowan for helping her with the choices which she enjoyed very much.

This was followed by gelato which Carmen preferred to ice-cream.

After the meal they drove off to Bar Beach for a walk along the beach. Carmen was amazed at the amount of exposed female acreage just lying around on the beach even at this late hour in the evening. Such a sight would have attracted some serious kamikaze feats from males in India!

"I know I have not been here long Rowan but I have not seen any aboriginal people."

"No, they usually live in communities. I have sometimes seen some aboriginal patients when I pass by the renal department. Apparently they have chronic kidney disease possibly related to their high incidence of diabetes, poor nutrition, obesity, high blood pressure and lack of exercise and smoking etcetera."

"How are they as patients to modern medicine?"

"It is important to observe their cultural demands when dealing with them. I was told by a friend never to make direct eye contact. They can view that as being rude, disrespectful or even aggressive. To convey polite respect, the appropriate approach is to lower your eyes in conversation. If you don't comply they just don't turn up for future appointments."

"We as Indians also have our own cultural demands."

"And the British have their own too." Rowan added.

"What kind of work do the aboriginals usually do?" Carmen was interested.

"Many work as labourers on cattle ranches. Some still hunt and gather. Some live on the outskirts of towns and do some labour work in towns."

"It must be very hard to for them to accept their plight. We are lucky that in India the British did somewhat look after us even after they had satisfied their own needs."

"Well here, various attempts were made initially to eliminate the aboriginals completely. Almost a Hitlerian thought," Rowan continued.

"No. It seems Hitler may have got his idea from here," Carmen remarked.

"Did you know that some government policies of assimilation led to Aboriginal children being forcibly removed from their parents some years ago? These *Stolen Generations* as they are called were put in adoptive families and institutions and forbidden from speaking their native languages. Their names were often changed. Some of them were even sexually abused. Similar to when the British illegitimate children were shipped here aided by the blessings of the holy catholic church to do menial jobs in catholic institutions. They were also sexually abused by the clergy."

"That is truly disgraceful," Carmen commented.

"In spite of their individually professed invented and improvised noble breed, the average Australian is of a convict heritage. After the American war of independence, when America closed its doors to the British criminals they were all sent here. Some of their crimes were very petty," Rowan informed.

"Stealing apples? Like *Agustine of Hippo*?"

"The thinking brain of those in power in those days was different. Nevertheless, today there are two hundred and fifty distinct language groups in the aboriginal cultures."

"Good. Yet again however, we should let bygones be bygones"

"Unfortunately there are always a few people that can't and continue to stir. They have nothing else to occupy their lives."

The sea breezes were now beginning to push for recognition of their existence. However both Carmen and Rowan were not equipped to offer any resistance to the ensuing discomfort.

"I think we should go home mum. What do you think?"

"I agree."

They walked back to the car, each entertaining their own thoughts of gratitude.

Back at home, they decided to have some brandy.

"That was a wonderful evening Rowan. Thank you."

"Plenty more from where that came mum. I love you very much. And thank you for going through all you went through for me."

Both of them burst into tears. Both of them knew they were crying for grandma, Felicity.

"I should write to Cecil tomorrow and tell him about this wonderful evening we had." And thank you for suggesting the lasagne. That was very nice."

"No problem mum."

"I must try and make some lasagne at home," Carmen ventured

I think we should go to bed now."

"Alright. Goodnight."

"Goodnight"

Rowan had had a long day. He slept as soon as his head hit the pillow and was soon snoring. Carmen thought about the day's events for a while before succumbing to sleep herself.

26

Next morning after Rowan had gone off to the hospital, Carmen was left alone in the apartment. Her thoughts took over. She thought of the pleasant evening that she had with Rowan yesterday. She was also keen to meet James' family. Rowan had told her that they were quite a happy and delightful lot. She thought she would cook an Indian meal and invite them over. She would discuss this plan later with Rowan when he came back from the hospital.

"That is an excellent idea mum," Rowan agreed when he was informed about her plan, on his arrival home that evening.

"I will go very low on the spice. I don't want them to be upset by the food," Carmen said.

Together they shopped for the Indian condiments and ventured to Sydney to harvest some more. Carmen was determined to impress the Regans with her culinary talents and to that end would leave no stone unturned. Rowan was to invite them on the coming Saturday.

Meanwhile at the Regan's household, James decided to spill his secret with the girls.

"You self-centred bastard! All you men are bastards! I thought you were different. How could you desert a pregnant woman?" Fiona roared at him.

"So Rowan is our brother then. You should marry Carmen, dad. Then we can have a family again," Fatima saw an easy way out.

"Shut up," Faye interjected. Faye was already despising Carmen as she suspected that James may get interested in her and she may take her beloved mother's memory away from the house and her mother may be lost in oblivion. It did not seem like a good idea to Faye.

James sensed that Faye may create a problem in this matter.

"I have asked her but she has refused," James explained.

Faye appeared relieved.

"Does it surprise you?" Fiona continued.

"I am sorry. I was a different person then. All I ask of you at this stage is to be nice to her during her stay here."

"Yes we will," Fiona and Fatima recited in a chorus.

Faye refrained from any comment.

The penny also dropped for Fiona. She realised now why James was not keen on her showing any interest in Rowan after the Christmas party.

James realised he may have work to do with Faye. But Carmen had been adamant in her refusal. It is not going to happen. Need he even bother with Faye?

In the carpark at the DeCruz apartment their olfaction was intercepted by the flavours of Carmen's cooking, as they got out of their car. Faye had abstained from coming.

The girls deposited the flowers they had brought with Carmen and James provided Rowan with a bottle of Sauvignon Blanc.

"Where is your other sister?" Rowan inquired.

"Faye had to go somewhere," Fiona covered for Faye and then hugged Rowan.

Fatima ran forward and hugged Rowan and then Carmen.

"Dad has told us everything. Welcome to our family," Fatima spilt.

"Carmen, I think you must marry dad," Fiona inveigled straightaway. She had thought about the matter and her dad's dirty antics in those early times. She must let Carmen know that nothing stood in her way now.

James was flabbergasted. He was not expecting them to move so fast. But he hoped it may work.

Carmen appeared checkmated, "I need to think about it. This is not an easy decision for me."

"Dad was a bastard then, Carmen. But he has changed now," Fiona continued.

James and Rowan looked at each other and hugged.

"Let's celebrate today," Rowan interrupted," I have some Sauvignon Blanc from Bordeaux"

A pang ran through James' heart for Freida. That was her favourite wine too. They had shared many such bottles in those loving times. He argued within himself, Freida could never be here. Some things have to happen for other things to happen. In fact her absence allowed this to happen and in a sense he was pleased. With Freida around, this matter could have had a disastrous outcome although he knew that if Freida knew his past she would also baptise him as a bastard too.

James looked at Carmen closely and did find her attractive even now. She was wearing jeans and a top that exposed the medial fraction of her breasts, just enough to upset the balance of his sex hormones. He remembered his former bed encounters with her. He just hoped she would change her mind and very soon.

During the evening Fiona and Fatima obsequiously followed Carmen and helped with the kitchen agenda in spite of Carmen repeatedly hectoring them that they were the guests and she was the host. The girls were also beginning to understand Rowan and his ways very much better now.

The dinner party progressed brilliantly aided by the alcoholic beverages. Carmen had cooked *samosas, tandoori chicken, pork vindaloo, barramundi curry, pulao and* a *dodol* pudding for desert which went very well with the guests.

The girls were awed by Carmen's soft spoken accent and polite Indian manners.

"Carmen, you and Rowan have convinced me that I should visit India," Fiona began.

Rowan who initially wished she would forget the offer, now changed his mind.

"Indeed you should," Carmen replied.

"Yes you should," seconded Rowan.

"I want to go too," Fatima interjected.

"Of course," Rowan added.

"When you come to India, you must leave reality behind. There is no reality in India. I mean that in a complimentary sense," Carmen explained.

"I agree," James said.

"Yes. When you have time to think which is not often, questions will arise in your mind. The existence of god, the essence of people, the nature of the human mind, the soul etcetera. And then there will be questions about human free will. Can we really choose our destiny, or is everything that happens fated to happen?" It was obvious Rowan had been bothered with these issues in his time.

"And when you can't answer these questions and in the absence of science, a god awaits you," Fiona added.

"Some Indian gurus may even convince you that you as an individual do not exist at all," Carmen continued.

"And questions like, does the existence of the universe point to the existence of a god?" continued Rowan.

James was watching the conversation proceed and now contributed, "In all this, true wisdom is found in admitting ignorance. And as *Richard Feynman* whom I have mentioned to you girls before, put it, we must be open to the fact that we might be wrong and to changing our mind if we are."

"The concept of a soul helps to stitch the mind and brain together," Rowan continued.

"The soul is considered nonphysical and can exist without a body. Different religions believe that different things happen to the soul after death.

Christians believe that the soul goes to heaven or hell. Hindus believe the soul continues to find other bodies to inhabit till it achieves liberation. Islam believes the soul awaits the arrival of judgement day when its fate will be decided," Carmen explained.

"Everything that was once explained by the soul, like emotions, memories, personality etcetera is now explained by the activity of the brain, including activity in the limbic system, and the prefrontal cortex. There is nothing left for the soul to do and, hence there is no reason to suppose that it exists," James added.

Rowan felt relieved. From unreality the conversation was slowly getting towards reality.

"The philosophers have been busy bringing in new terms like dualism, eliminativism etcetera to explain this. Terms which only perhaps hopefully at least the individual philosopher only understands," Carmen added.

James thought that if Carmen changes her mind in his favour, she would provide him excellent argumentation for his own philosophical sojourns.

It was getting late and James decided it was time to go home.

"Girls, I think we should be moving," James began.

"That was a wonderful evening Carmen, thank you so much for inviting us," Fiona said.

"Yes thank you very much. I especially like the pork vindi stuff," Fatima said.

"Yes Carmen, I had no idea you could cook so well," James added.

"No problem. I am so glad you enjoyed it James," Carmen replied.

"And thank you for suggesting *Feynman*, I have to look him up," Rowan finished.

When the Regans left, Rowan congratulated his mother, "You did very well there today, mum."

"Yes I am very pleased it went well."

"The ball is in your court now, mum."

"What do you mean?"

"To be or not to be married to James."

"Once bitten twice shy."

"Yes, but it was not entirely his fault."

Carmen understood where he was coming from. She had misled him and instigated it herself. She was not repentant.

She needed to think about it tonight and tomorrow and the day after tomorrow and the day after, if need be. She also realised that Rowan would know the exact truth from the Reagan girls sooner or later. How James had deserted her in her pregnancy. She decided she will deal with that, when and if that eventuates.

'Carmen, Carmen, Carmen it is', was the conversation in the Reagan car, on the way home.

"I love her red lipstick," Fatima observed.

"Yes I used to have a few shirts stained with that lipstick in those days," James responded.

"She must have really loved you dad and I think she still does," Fiona added.

"I think so too. I can tell by the way she looks at

you dad," Fatima mentioned.

Only James was not so sure. He only hoped that Carmen would soon provide a propitious decision.

Next day it was decided by James, Fiona and Fatima that Rowan and Carmen be invited over for an quasi Irish dinner soon at their Charlestown home. Faye remained quiet. Finally when the die appeared almost cast, she spoke, "Can you not take them to a restaurant?"

"You just have to meet her. You will change your mind," Fatima said.

"Yes. First meet her and then make up your mind," Fiona added.

Faye was not impressed and left the room hurriedly. In her room she remembered her darling mother Freida and wept. Faye was the sensitive one and the one closest to Freida. She thought for a short while and as if implored by Freida's spirit to take care of dad, realised that her dad seems much happy now than for the many months after Freida's funeral. Should I spoil it for him? I will never be able to forgive myself.

She came back to them and explained, "I am sorry. I am prejudging Carmen even before meeting her. I will cooperate with whatever you plan. I love you dad. Count mc in."

James was pleased with her response. Only one more hurdle to go. Carmen's decision.

Carmen woke up late next morning after Rowan had left for the hospital for his rounds. He left a note that he would not be home for lunch. After a minimal breakfast Carmen decided to go for a walk and set her mind working on the problem at hand.

The streets were deserted. She wondered if it was a day of national mourning.

She was mainly interested in the cons rather than the pros of a 'yes' decision for James. Could she trust James again with all his sweet ways? Something very deep within her said 'no'. If she agreed it would only be for convenience. She could stay here in Australia. She would have a much better life and Rowan would also be greatly benefited in his career ambitions. She felt she was still attracted to James and could get into bed with him if sanctioned. Would she orgasm? She did not know. There was no 'try before you buy' option available this time. She had already exhausted her 'fly now pay later' plan option with Rowan's birth.

As she was walking along she recognised the priest she had met recently coming from the opposite direction. He appeared not to be aware of the obstacles on the footpath presented by the non-sentient objects.

"Good morning father," she greeted him.

The poor priest was confused. He could not recollect where he had seen this face before. But as the call of duty demands, to never refuse a chance to proselytize a soul he responded, "Hello, how are you?"

Carmen was in two minds whether to discuss her current problem with him and ask for advice. She remembered her encounter with Father Joseph Carvalho. Could she ever trust a priest? Their only function to her appeared to be to make excuses for god's mistakes, with certain well-rehearsed and fixed recitations. That failing, they invent lies.

The priest was still trying to work out where he had seen this face before. Could it be in Singapore where he had holidayed about a month ago? That was where he last saw a lot of coloured faces.

"I am good. I am sorry I could not attend Mass this morning", Carmen replied.

The penny dropped for him. This was the mother of the plastic surgeon.

"You must confess your sins at confession, not on the road here. We have confessions on Wednesdays and Saturday afternoons. I will see you at confession."

"Okay. Bye Father."

"Bye."

Confession was the last thing on her mind. What did she have to confess? It was not like when she was a child and an obligatory weekly confession was imposed on her and Cecil by her mother, Felicity. She remembered those times when she had to make up some sins just to fulfil Felicity's mandatory requirements.

As she walked along she noticed that some eateries were beginning to demonstrate their lunch time utility by providing their own territorial odours to entice the passers-by. She wanted to try a meat pie as suggested by Rowan in an earlier conversation. She ventured into a shop and asked for a pie. The morbidly ultra-rotund factotum lady behind the counter was dressed in black and had a broomstick in her hand. The lady recited a series of options available and demanded a firmer choice from her. Carmen finally ordered a steak and kidney pie from amongst the other greek accented choices. The lady was quick to pack the pie in a brown paper bag and demanded payment. The lady had encountered changing Indians minds on several occasions before. Carmen paid and walked home with her lunch choice.

The ambient air at home was hot and she summoned the air conditioner to aid. As the temperature cooled she reached for some of yesterday's left over wine in the fridge and poured herself a glass. She sipped it slowly lubricating the meat pie as it found its way.

The wine soon took effect. She needed to lie down.

She thought about James. She felt really sorry for him. She wished his wife was alive. Three girls to manage without a mother. It must be very difficult.

Soon she fell asleep.

She was woken up by the shrieking screams of a sulphur-crested cockatoo just outside. It took her a second to recognise her whereabouts but she soon realised that the unpleasant sound of the bird easily gave the continent away. Somehow the birds in this country are not vocally gifted she thought. However she had her own task on hand. Should she volunteer herself to James to help him out? Would that be the moral thing to do considering his position? Also she really did not want to go back to Byculla. She really did not want Rowan to go back to Byculla also. It seemed obvious to her that she may have to accept a non-Indian bride for Rowan. But then she could always import an Indian bride. Such brides come with a vast dowry. For how many more generations could this importing of brides continue? She was a forward thinking woman. She had also noted that Rowan was beginning to lose some of his Indian identity already.

When she was in Bombay, Cecil had told her that there was a goan lady doctor, Loretta Pimento in his apartment building who may be a good match for Rowan when he returns back from Australia. Loretta had qualified as a specialist gastroenterologist and was aware of Rowan. Rowan also had heard of her. However nothing was worked out between the families yet.

Back here, so far the two Reagan girls who came along to dinner appeared to like her although she had not met the last one. It seemed odd to her that one did not come. Keeping away is often a sign of dissent. Carmen was not sure. She would take her own time to make this decision. Or as her father, Porfiro used to say, 'never jump from the frying pan into the fire'.

Her thoughts now raced to cooking for tonight. There was some lamb marinating in yogurt salt, ginger, and garlic in the fridge that she had planned to cook in a *biryani*. She knew Rowan would like that very much. She had all the required spices, cardamom, cinnamon, and mace, and the fresh herbs, cilantro and mint, saffron threads and turmeric to add the bright hues of orange to the long-grain basmati rice. She remembered how the custom officials were kind enough to help. Also with their recent shopping spree they had collected rosewater and pandan water. She remembered she even had the aluminium foil.

She set to work. Soon the kitchen acquired the odours of the *biryani* and the passing flies attempted to join the feast. Luckily their incursions were restricted by the flyscreens so they hovered outside pleading discrimination.

Rowan came home a bit later and was pleased with Carmen's efforts. He opened a bottle of Sauvignon Blanc and they settled down to appease their hunger.

During the meal Rowan informed Carmen that the Reagans had invited them over next Saturday for dinner and he had accepted.

The conversations were next limited to Carmen's experiences of the day.

Eventually Rowan announced that he was tired and wanted to go to bed.

Carmen sat up for a while. She had more thinking to do.

27

Carmen and Rowan arrived at the Regan house at Charlestown as scheduled. Carmen was awed and could not hold her admiration, "You girls have a very beautiful home here."

"You should come and share it with us," Fiona replied looking at Carmen and waiting patiently for an answer.

Carmen realised she had put her foot in her mouth. She smiled not wanting to give herself away. She had thought about it. James had been kind to her. But he had also been very kind to her in India before she got pregnant. It was after she got pregnant that he had chameleoned. She remembered *Shakespeare*, *'The evil that men do lives after them; The good is oft interred with their bones*.' She felt her body could take him as he was still attractive to her but the spirit was still very very unwilling. She adored the girls. But they were James' girls. They would of course go with him in case of a problem. She knew Rowan would care for her always. She could rely on Rowan here. She should have talked to Rowan before they came. She felt the matter would resurface tonight. She should have come prepared.

Faye who was good at doing little but usually full of ideas for others refrained from any remarks this time.

And Fatima smiled placidly.

Noting her embarrassment James intervened, "Leave her alone girls. Only she can make that decision and she may need time to change her mind. No one will talk about it tonight. Agreed? Carmen you just enjoy yourself tonight."

James and the girls were perfect hosts.

The evening started with cream sherry and merlot wines. Nuts, olives, cheeses and other delicacies were already set in bowls on the table.

For dinner the girls served *colcannon*, an Irish favourite with mashed potatoes and beans and sausages. Potato candy with peanut butter and ground sugar were served as desert.

Coffee and port followed.

"It is interesting. I was just wondering how different peoples and cultures have different foods. Take Indian food. Take Irish food," Fatima started.

It was obvious that the conversation would revolve around food with Fatima's recent interjection.

"The story of the evolution of food is a long one Fatima. It starts with what is locally available in the region, the local trade, the local religion, the local culture, colonialism etcetera," James began.

"Yes. We initially started as hunter gatherers. Then the agricultural revolution took place in the Fertile Crescent, what is today Iraq, Syria, eastern Turkey, Lebanon, and Israel. This led to the domestication of plants and animals, like goats, sheep, and cows. From there, agriculture next travelled to Greece, then to

Italy, eastern Spain, and central Germany and finally reached southern Britain," Rowan contributed. He was being introduced to the Reagan type discussions and appeared to love such argumentation.

"It is also amazing how each culture has a staple starch. Being rice in Asia, corn in Mesoamerica which was initially populated by the American Indians, potatoes and quinoa in South America, sorghum in Africa, and teff in Ethiopia," Carmen added.

"What is teff Carmen? I'd like to try some," Fatima inquired.

"Sorry Fatima you can't, teff is a type of grass grown in Africa. It is ground and fermented to make a flat bread," Carmen continued.

"The American Indians had their own crops with maize, squash, beans, tomatoes, chilis, amaranth, cactus, avocado and guava," Rowan added

"Africa gave the world watermelons, beans, okra, cola nuts, tamarind, palms, finger millet, black-eyed peas, sorghum and yam," Carmen remembered.

"Initially there were also dietary restrictions associated with religions. The Hebrew Jews are particularly interesting. They invented rituals to define behaviour by members of their group, to bring them under the authority of those in power and create cooperation among the group. In the initial stage there was only one dietary restriction imposed. Humans could not eat blood. Hebrews thought that blood contained the life of the creature, and all life belongs to God. The blood prohibition is still in effect among Jews; animals have to be slaughtered painlessly and the blood completely drained to be kosher. According to their god, Hebrews can eat anything with a cloven hoof and that chews its cud like goats, sheep, and cows but not animals that have only one or the other, like the camel that chews its cud but has toes, nor the pig that has cloven hooves but doesn't chew its cud. And among people who keep kosher, it has come to be interpreted as meaning that you can never mix any milk and meat products in the same meal," James continued.

The girls were listening very intently. This was very interesting they thought.

"Then humans invented fermentation and a whole series of new foods, including bread, wine and beer, cheese, and pickled or cured vegetables and fruits appeared," Rowan continued.

"I heard that true restaurants appeared first in Paris in the mid-18th century," Faye added.

"Yes, providing the subject for some of Renoir's famous paintings," James said.

"You mean *Luncheon of the Boating Party* and *Lunch at The Restaurant Fournaise*," Fiona added. She loved Renoir's work.

"Exactly," James replied.

Not wanting to be outdone on the Indian front Carmen added, "The religion introduced by the Aryans who came to India from the north forms the basis of Hinduism, based on the *Rigveda* in Sanskrit, which is one of the oldest religious texts in existence. When the Aryan gods were failing with the widespread famine, drought, and wars throughout

India, the Brahmans which is the highest caste, began to be the object of suspicion and anger from the lower classes began to show. The Brahmans decided to reinvent themselves to survive, so they began to add new sacred writings with food prohibitions particularly to denote who could eat with whom, and also to forbid cow eating. They came forward as ascetic, celibate, and vegetarian."

"That is interesting Carmen," Faye commented.

"Yes now you know why hindus do not eat beef," Rowan said.

"In Europe, in very early times the Venetians monopolized the spice trade. In the spice wars that followed, the French beat the Venetians, the English beat the French and finally the British Empire was brought into existence," James continued.

"Yes. The Portuguese and Spanish were the first in the colonisation business, but were muscled out later by England, the Netherlands, and France," Rowan provided.

The conversation was getting very informative for the girls particularly with every new contribution. They were also learning some spicy European history.

Carmen continued, "The Portuguese sent Vasco da Gama who, made it all the way to Calicut on the west coast of India, where he came in contact with Asian ships from Malacca. The Portuguese conquered Calicut, destroyed the rival Muslim fleets under Alfonso de Albuquerque, and set up a military post in India. They soon took Goa where I come from, which remained a port colony until this century. The Portuguese took over Malacca on the Malay Peninsula and Macao in China, and they had a foothold in Japan for a while. When the Japanese emperor realised that the accompanying Jesuits had a plan they were immediately ordered to leave. The Portuguese set up posts in Java, Sumatra, and throughout Indonesia which is where the spices come from."

"Is that why goans have Portuguese surnames?" Fatima inquired.

"Yes, Goa being a Portuguese colony, the Portuguese culture was forced on the local inhabitants," Carmen informed.

"Nowadays all over the world we have a new culture of wealthy, overweight, middle-and upper-class women, who want to eat a simple diet as a way to lose weight and become sort of spiritually purified," James laughed

"That's actually true of most food ideologies nowadays, even in India. They promise that if you eat a certain way, you will be healthy, moral, politically correct and a better person. They're a lot like religions in that way; they require a conversion and complete commitment," Rowan added.

"May be we need a new religion. The traditional ones are not working," Fiona joked.

"Exactly so," Faye echoed.

"Also immigration affects food habits. In the last century about sixty million people left Europe and went to North and South America, Australia, and New Zealand. The population of North America went from six million to eighty million, largely due to immigration. In these circumstances the food began to include multi-culture ingredients providing a newer taste," James said.

"You mean there were no immigration quotas in those days?" Faye asked.

"Yes perhaps there were. But it would seem that the quotas would depend on the labour and other requirements of the immigrating country," Rowan helped.

"Apparently studies show that the first generation to emigrate rarely becomes fully assimilated, but their children, the second generation, who are born in the new country, want to assimilate. Ironically, it's the third generation that struggles to figure out who they are and where they came from and gets interested in the old language, culture, and recipes," James continued.

"So really what should we be doing dad since we have already past the third generation?" Faye asked.

"You are now fully Australian my dear," James said.

"Isn't it interesting that India and Australia were close to each other at the South Pole when the Earth was once a supercontinent called Pangea? Then the Indian tectonic plate moved northwards and collided with the Eurasian Plate, to cause the Himalayas," Rowan attempted the Australia-India connection.

"Yes we learnt in school that when plates slide past

one another, it is called a transform boundary, as in the San Andreas Fault. When plates move apart from each other, it is called a divergent boundary, as in the mid-atlantic range. And when two plates are moving toward each other, it is called a convergent boundary. If a plate is dense enough, then it can descend below the other, into the mantle, as in around the Pacific Plate-New Zealand and Japan. Regions where plates descend back into the Earth are known as subduction zones. That is why volcanoes are found all along the rim of the Pacific Plate, where subduction is occurring," Faye remembered.

"It is an interesting world and we are so lucky to be living at this time," James added.

"The people that come after us will be even more luckier," Fatima predicted.

"Not necessarily. Not with all the nuclear weaponry we have today," James said.

The girls and particularly Faye were very impressed by Carmen's knowledge.

"You know so much Carmen," Faye observed.

"I learnt that from your dad. Give up small talk and read as much as possible. The more you read, the more you remember. And never be selfish with knowledge," Carmen informed.

James smiled. A bonus point for him. Things may be looking up he thought.

"Indian food is so tasty. I want you to teach me to cook Indian food. When can we start?" Faye pleaded.

"Me too," Fatima continued.

"And don't forget me," Fiona did not want to miss out.

"Carmen since you have a few cooking recruits, this calls for more drinks. Anyone?" James asked.

"I will pass. I need to drive," Rowan said.

Carmen and the girls opted for brandy.

"What you said today was very interesting Carmen. Thank you," Fatima said.

"Plenty more from where that came from," Carmen smiled.

James was beginning to feel a bit hopeful but he was still not sure.

The girls, Carmen and Rowan got on well tonight. He felt that it may all be alcohol induced. Anyhow at least it was a beginning.

The evening ended well and after the usual 'byes' the DeCruzes left for home. Carmen and Rowan discussed the event as Rowan drove home.

"The girls are really very lovely," Carmen commented.

"I told you so mum," Rowan replied.

"I do really like them all."

"The eldest Fiona is very nice to me," Rowan reminisced.

"I am very tempted to marry James. What do you think?"

"Although the decision should entirely be yours, I think so too. But I will support you, whichever way you go."

"Well, he can't go away anywhere now and there's no Rowan in my tummy and this is not Byculla. What can go wrong?"

"Yeah. I think so too. Think about it."

"No. I don't need I really need to think any further. I can't go wrong this time."

"Whatever it is, it's finally your own decision."

"I will accept his offer. When you go to work tomorrow can you ask James to come over? I don't want you to be around."

"I understand."

Next day when James arrived, Carmen was ready, "I have decided to marry you James for better only, but not for worse. Will you accept?"

James was overjoyed. He now had it straight from the horse's mouth.

"When? Tomorrow?" he remembered his first proposal from the paediatric patient in Leeds. Maybe not at that time, but somehow now, those days in Leeds were good days, he thought.

"Okay," Carmen replied.

"Settled. We need to celebrate your decision Carmen. The girls will also be very happy. What do you say, we all go out for Chinese tonight? I will book for seven o'clock tonight"

"That would be good. I will inform Rowan. He will be happy too."

They met at a restaurant at New Lambton. The restaurant was not crowded so the owner could devote all his attention to these few customers.

"Carmen you don't know how happy I am that you have decided in favour of dad," Fiona admitted.

"You need to wish me well," Carmen laughed.

"More than that," Faye added.

"I always like a good deal. Thank you Carmen," Fatima added.

"Some things have to happen, darling," Carmen responded.

James smiled at Carmen with an, 'I think I love you' look.

Carmen reciprocated with a similar look.

The others resorted to *Robert Browning*'s, "*God's in His heaven, all's right with the world*" looks.

The choices on the menu were galore. Rowan was suffering a choice paralysis. This feeling was not new to him. From past experience, he had learnt to always restrict his choices to the same every time. This eliminated the trauma of making a wrong decision and also saved time. As a younger person particularly when he had to choose ice cream flavours, he had worked out that when he chose a flavour, he always felt he should have got the other one leaving him repentant for the rest of the day. To overcome the feeling he always stayed with one flavour. In fact at medical school he remembered how his friends chided him that he had the tendency of a monogamist. He personally saw nothing wrong with that.

So he sat back and let the others make their choices. Likewise James also watched.

It was a women only ordering day. Faye and Fatima opted for *sweet corn and chicken soup* to start. The others abstained from soup.

Spring rolls, curried puffs and *steam pork dumplings* for entrees were next followed by *Bombay chicken, Balinese seafood, honey king prawns, sweet and sour pork spare ribs, Mongolian lamb, Thai red curried duck, Masaman curried beef* and fried rice.

James chose a chardonnay to grace the occasion.

With the gluttonous task at hand there was no time

for any conversation except for expressions of delight as the meal proceeded. It was an enjoyable evening for all.

Next day James got to work on the marriage civil registration matters and was scrupulous in fulfilling every requirement and the marriage took place in about one months time. The celebration was intentionally limited to the family to include James' parents, Janet and her husband Michael Dougherty who was a police officer and their daughters, Cathy and Amanda. James' office girls and their partners were also invited.

The ceremony was held at the Reagan household and the lady celebrant was instructed to speed the proceedings as much as possible. However as all celebrants need to see, hear, smell, taste and feel their own humour as the best available around, no amount of bribery would have helped and the celebrant did exactly as she was told not to do. Carmen would have preferred a church wedding. She knew James would not be keen on that. She also knew she may not eligible as per the infallible catholic canon laws with which she always seemed to have a conflictual relationship in spite of her repeated attempts at signing a peace treaty.

James had prebooked at a restaurant in town for the celebrations. All the attendees had a wonderful time. At least they said so, on departing.

James and Carmen spent the wedding night at a hotel. Sex was high on the agenda after a few drinks. Carmen was anxious. However with James in charge, she had no difficulty and although her recurred catholic theist mental faculties provide an initial barrier, this was soon overcome. Old times were back again! Life is for living! Life is not to prepare for an imaginary afterlife, she thought again.

28

As expected Carmen and Rowan moved into the Reagan household at Charlestown, much to the Regans' delight.

Apart from a study desk and chair and his bed, Rowan's room was also equipped with a bookcase which was soon weighed down with his massive collection of books relating to varied subjects and of varying dimensions and binding from paperbacks to hard covers. When he lived at the hospital resident quarters, he often strolled down Hunter Street in his free time, visiting the many bookshops and spending time in there, seeking books that may often have left him with an attack of monetarypenia. His need for knowledge was obsessive. In this respect he was almost a replica of James again. He also had an excellent memory which he was often surprised with himself. He could recollect facts vividly from books he had read in primary school. These facts presented to him, just like that, on the spur of the moment. His interests also were wide and multiple, ranging from deep sea scuba diving monsters to the benefits of a nuclear war. Rowan provided a continuous source of information for the girls. For them, there was never a dull moment with Rowan around. All the girls too were equipped with very inquisitive and questioning minds. In this regard both Freida and James had provided similar encouragement to them in their formative years.

Fiona liked Rowan as a brother and also did not like him as a brother as he would have suited her romantic interests perfectly and she was particularly attracted to his looks and his Indian accent. She was very slowly getting to accept him as her own sibling. The other girls adored him. They loved his gentlemanly ways and were glad just to have a brother whose knowledge of some subjects was very enviable.

One evening when the family was gathered after dinner Fiona asked him, "What kind of music do you like Rowan?" The earlier these idiosyncrasies are sorted out, the better the assimilation and lesser the disagreements, Fiona had deciphered.

"I like all music Fiona but I love jazz most of all."

"Jazz, wow, I love it too," voiced James in the vicinity.

"Everybody loves jazz. It belongs to our period," Carmen added.

"I did some very interesting reading on jazz some time ago," Rowan announced.

"Tell us about it," Fatima as usual, was curious.

"It all started before the American civil war, when African rhythms and European form were combined into a dance craze which was taken up by the African slaves. It was called the 'cakewalk'. The slaves of the south in America used to gather for their cakewalk competitions regularly. Here they ridiculed their masters' dancing with arched backs and high stepping. This music slowly evolved into ragtime which added syncopation."

"What is syncopation?" Fatima wanted to know.

"Syncopation is when the normal flow of rhythm is interrupted unexpectedly. It is something that disrupts your expectation. When you are expecting a certain rhythm you are surprised by an unexpected one," Rowan explained rolling his tongue. He continued, "Ragtime then evolved into Dixieland jazz. Dixieland jazz used syncopation and improvisation in newer ways."

"What is improvisation?" Fatima asked.

"Improvisation come from improvise. You know that. Making up on the spur of the moment. It is the immediate creation of a melody on the spot. There is no preparation. Improvisation meant not only changing the melody of a given piece but sometimes turning a mistake into an unexpected advantage."

"Very clever," Fatima commented.

"I do it all the time in my conversations, if I find I have put my foot into my mouth," Fiona joked.

"Improvising is often compared to storytelling. Improvisers use vocabulary to tell a story when they create a solo, increasing the interest as the solo progresses through a variety of musical notes," Rowan explained.

"Interesting," Faye commented.

"Dixieland jazz grew out of the lively march that marked a New Orleans funeral. It relied mainly on the marching instruments like the banjo and tuba. The seriousness of these funerals usually progressed to happy dancing with the extremes of grief and joy both present in the ceremony," Rowan continued.

James was listening intently, "To me, eventually it seems the line between ragtime and jazz is a very fuzzy one."

"These are really evolution distinctions and bound

to have fuzzy lines," Carmen intervened.

"The blues began as a sad expression of emotion. To play the blues is to release pent-up feelings. Think of Ray Charles and Sam Cooke nowadays," Rowan went on.

"The blues are really a way of reminding oneself that any problem could be worse." Carmen laughed.

"Because the early slaves were not allowed to travel, white performers who heard them took advantage of their inspiration and transported their music across the United States. You will remember black-face minstrelsy with the "Black and White Minstrel Shows," Rowan continued.

"They're great. I used to love them. The show was very popular," James said.

"I loved them too." Carmen agreed.

"Do you know how the word jazz originated Rowan? It is an interesting word," James asked.

"I really can't say for sure. But I read that in the cakewalk contest the winner was declared the *chaise beau* which literally means, 'the man who sat on the throne'. Then this was altered to jazzbo, which was later shortened to jazz."

"That's interesting Rowan, thanks," James was happy with the explanation.

"Swing evolved from this almost at the same time. Swing combined syncopation with improvisation and arrangement. Boogie-woogie which is a heavy-handed but highly rhythmic style soon followed. Then Bebop was born, and so were *Dizzy Gillespie* and *Miles Davis*. Boogie-woogie was a precursor of rock and roll. Then with the invention of the microphone, *Bing Crosby* and *Frank Sinatra* and *Pat Boone* shot into the limelight.

"So jazz, in sum, is syncopation and improvisation," Fiona understood.

"Right," Rowan replied.

"That's very interesting Rowan. Goans really know their music well don't they?" James complimented Rowan.

"Dad, do you mind? Go on Rowan," Fatima was not finished listening.

"Sorry Fatima," James apologised for interrupting.

"Can you please continue with the history Rowan?" Fatima persisted.

"Not much more Fatima. A chain reaction followed. Cool jazz was a reaction to bebop. In time came 'modal' jazz which used ancient church scales and then 'fusion' jazz, which is a jazz and rock blend. Nowadays we have 'free' jazz. Free jazz has no set chord changes but there is a constant tempo with spontaneous improvisation and no rules. Some musicians went back to the blues to make 'soul' jazz. This relies mainly on the marching instruments like the banjo and tuba. And really that's all there is to the story"

"That was most interesting Rowan thank you for sharing," Fiona was now competently informed about jazz. She could now enjoy it better, she thought. The brilliant creators!

"As I said before, in jazz, the melodies can be pre-composed in advance or improvised on the spot. The pre-composed melody is called 'head'. I hope that was enough of a shell?" Rowan finished.

"The improvisation is called the tail?" Fatima joked.

"No, no. It stays improvisation. The front line of jazz groups consists of trumpet, saxophone, and trombone. When front line players are playing together, they are often playing the pre-composed melody. The rhythm section consists of drums, bass, piano, with or without a guitar. The rhythm section usually plays continuously throughout a performance, as opposed to the front line players."

"Seems like the rhythm section also provides the beat, isn't it?" Faye asked.

"Yes. The rhythm section provides rhythmic feel, form, and harmony. Rhythm section playing requires very good teamwork," Rowan informed.

"I suppose what contributes to our perceptions of a music piece is essentially the tempo, the volume, and how the music ends," James commented.

"Yes. It seems a fast tempo and loud volume would make us happy and excited and sometimes possibly aggressive. A slow tempo and low volume would make us melancholy and down," Fiona observed.

"That is correct. Have you heard of gypsy rock and *Django Reinhardt*?" Rowan asked.

"Who's that?" Fatima was curious.

"Well when *Louis Armstrong*, the jazz king, as you might know him, went to Europe, he met a chap called Django Reinhardt, who had only the index and middle fingers on his left hand. Playing together they both gave birth to gypsy rock."

"What happened to his fingers?" Fatima wanted to know.

"He lost the fingers putting out a fire in the caravan

his family lived in," Rowan explained.

"What does gypsy rock sound like?" Fiona inquired.

"I can't explain it in words. Everyone's music is very subjective and personal Fiona. To me it is great. It makes me feel good," Rowan replied.

"That's good Rowan. Thank you. I must listen to some gypsy rock," Fatima concluded.

"Yes. Me too. Thanks Rowan," Fiona added.

"Thanks," Faye repeated.

"In the context of your last remark James, its not only goans, but music itself is really a primal human condition isn't it? It is really an effortless and instinctive exercise in all of us. We could have possibly had an adaptive need for music. It does arouse great emotions of tenderness, love, triumph, and also fervour for war. Doesn't it? I get very 'touchy feely' when I listen to Edith Piaf," Rowan continued.

"Me too. I like listening to her," Carmen volunteered.

"In birds, singing is used to attract a mate or to defend a territory," Fiona, the bird sage added.

"*Charles Darwin* felt that music evokes such strong and complex emotions in us because it once served a function in human life similar to its function for birds namely a function in finding a mate. Music activates ancient, primal emotions in us because of its role in the emotionally charged business of attracting and defending a mate," James had read Darwin's, *On the Origin of Species*.

"Darwin felt that music had a role in human life

before we had language. His idea was a sort of 'musical protolanguage', a songlike communication system that is simpler than music as we know it today but it came before the evolution of full-blown speech. In other words, song came before speech in human evolution," Rowan had also read Darwin.

"Yes. With music there seems to be a tendency to share a similar emotional state, to sense a real connection to the people around you and to the identify with the message that the music projects. It has been used in church hymns, gospel music, national anthems, or concerts where people gather to make or hear music that they love," James mentioned.

"I would like to offer a motherly point of view. As human babies have an unusually long period of dependence on their mothers, mothers and babies need to communicate long before the babies can speak. Even though babies don't understand words, human mothers use sound to communicate and stay connected to their babies, which is again unlike other primates. May be again it was an evolutionary need for us," Carmen had made her maternal contribution.

Faye thought of how Freida used to sing the song 'How much is that doggie in the window?' to her as a baby. To choke her threatening tears and divert the conversation from turning to other mother child relationships, Faye offered, "Music is a group activity. It's common for groups of people to come together to make or listen to music at the same time. And when people do this, there is a sharing of a similar emotional state, to sense a real connection to the people around you as we do in music concerts."

"Also, there is always conflict between groups of people and this conflict can reduce a group's ability to deal with challenges from the environment or from other groups. Groups in which members cooperate can beat groups where individuals behave more selfishly and this cooperative behaviour can be achieved by music," James offered at this stage.

"That's why footy teams have their own anthems," Fatima worked out.

"Humans also get a lot of pleasure out of music. Maybe it was our need for pleasure also," Faye contributed.

"I know what I want for my next birthday," Fatima syncopated unexpectedly.

"Allow me. Let me improvise what your wish," Rowan replied.

"Go ahead"

"A Django Reinhardt CD"

"Ouch. You hit the nail right into my head!"

"We shall remember," Rowan smiled.

"To me music really seems like a human universal, but it's also tremendously diverse in its structure and meaning across cultures and time," Fiona recommenced.

"Ah, here it is important to distinguish between music and musicality. Music is really a social and cultural construct that shows the historical context in which it is created whereas musicality is the mental process that underlies our musical behaviour and perception, and these are much more stable across time and place. Musicality may also be found some other species," Rowan continued.

"Songbirds, humming birds, parrots, dolphins, whales, gibbons you mean?" Fiona added.

'Yes exactly. But their musicality is instinctive. Human musicality is learnt," Rowan explained.

"So as you say, the structure of the songs we produce depends on the cultural and historical context in which we are and not on genes we inherited from our parents," Fiona continued.

"I suppose learning one's songs through experience is a hallmark of human music. It sets us apart from other singing animals," James said. Freida should have been here tonight, he thought. She may have contributed more to this comparative music talk. He immediately called in the reality of the moment and let that thought vanish. He had learnt to do that quite confidently to survive his present reality.

"Humans might be the only animals that speak, but we are not the only animals that sing. Right?" Fatima asked.

"This time you hit the nail right on it's head," Rowan laughed.

"Nowadays of course we also have music therapy in which music is used to actively support people as they try to improve their well-being. It also lessens the impact of depression and anxiety and is also used in behavioural problems," Carmen introduced.

"If you ever have to use it on me please don't use Hindu chanting or very loud music," James laughed.

"Yes. Some music can trigger strong reactions or evoke bad memories which could very painful to some people," Rowan said.

"Did you have any bad experience with Hindu chanting dad?" Fatima asked.

"Chanting generally irritates me, including the Muslim call for prayers or the latin masses. I would rather listen to Frank Sinatra. Thanks."

"Yes, therapists have to be very careful in choosing the music. Sometimes it may leave the patient worse," Carmen offered.

"Incidentally, the top genre for depressed listeners is rock, followed closely by bebop. On the other end of the spectrum, blues is the least popular genre for people hoping to improve their moods," Rowan added.

"That seems obvious to me," Carmen said.

"What about classical music? How does that feature?" James asked.

"Classical music helps you focus. Music that has a tempo of sixty beats per minute increases the efficiency of the brain in processing information. The best way to use it is to have it playing softly in the background as you get on with your scheduled tasks," Rowan informed.

"Why sixty beats?" Faye asked.

"We feel a beat most strongly when the rate of beats is between about fifty and one hundred and fifty beats per minute. In that range, there seems to be a preference for a tempo of about one hundred beats per minute. This range is not radically different from the range of the human heartbeat, so it is intuitive to think that the musical beat has its origins in basic physiological rhythms like the heartbeat," Rowan explained.

Suddenly Fiona got up from her seat. She looked tired," I'm afraid I must beat it to sleep now."

She wished everyone, "*Bonne nuit*" and burst into song as she marched out of the room. She just did not have the vocal energy to improvise,

"*Allons enfant de la patrie Le jour de gloire est arrive....*'.

"It was a long and very interesting conversation. Thank you Rowan," James ended.

"Nothing big at the hospital tomorrow. So its okay," Rowan replied.

Everyone was yawning and ready for sleep. The requisite goodnights were exchanged while individual song favourites were being played in the individual minds.

29

One Sunday morning, well ensconced now in his new residence at Charlestown and aided by the absence of utility at the hospital, Rowan forced his presence to the window in the lounge. The sun may have travelled faster from the horizon and had already covered a significant part of its planned expedition of the hemisphere for the day. The clouds preferred to be cloister phobic.

Rowan spotted a bird with long legs crossing the road that he had never seen before. Though not a keen bird watcher himself, this bird was claiming his entire attention. He marvelled at its slow majestic stride across.

"What bird is that?" he needed to know.

Fatima and Fiona, both of whom, were also devoid of any current function and who were also present in the room jumped up and ran to the window to share his view. Both of them were avid bird watchers and loved any opportunity available to challenge their knowledge on the subject.

"That's a masked lapwing," Fatima identified.

"Notice it has spikes on the front end of its wings," Fiona contributed.

"Yes and it walks in a peculiar manner as if it owns the whole road," Rowan observed. His interest was aroused.

"The spikes are used against its predators," Fiona continued.

"Do you know birds are the only remnants of dinosaurs we have left today?" Rowan tried to interest himself further.

"Interesting isn't it? We still have some remnant dinosaur companions today," Fiona replied.

Bird knowledge was Fiona's hobby territory and she was not going to let this opportunity to impress Rowan pass by. This interest, and generally interest in nature itself had been inculcated in the Reagan girls both by James and Freida who took every opportunity to feed the young hungry minds. Fiona had been an ardent bird watcher herself for a very long time, often joining in bird watching group excursions with Fatima and Faye. She enjoyed reading everything about birds and was always obsessed by their genius. She always felt that, we as humans had a lot to learn from birds. Fatima and Faye also maintained a vivid interest in birds. And now they almost have a new recruit in Rowan. Bird watching could gain more momentum in the household if they could also provoke Rowan to get enthusiastic.

"What fascinates me most about birds is their capacity to orient and navigate and migrate. I have always been impressed by that," Rowan expressed his interest into birding.

"Many other animals also have an innate homing ability like bees, ants, salmon and even mice. Apparently birds orient by using magnetic fields, visual landmarks, sun and stars," Fiona informed.

"Birds aren't the only animals that migrate. The

seasonal migration of African mammals over the Serengeti is apparently a spectacular sight. Squid, salamanders, bats, and butterflies are also migratory," Fatima continued.

"It would be lovely to watch the Serengeti migration," Rowan said.

"But only from a very very safe distance," Fiona replied.

"I have watched it on film," Fatima said.

"I have seen it on film too. It is a magnificent sight," Fiona expressed her delight.

"Apparently in Canada people assemble to watch the annual salmon migration," Rowan informed.

"I have read about it. Apparently its a celebratory event there," Fiona added.

"Birds are very intelligent isn't it Fiona?" Rowan continued.

"It can't be insulting anymore to be accused of having a bird brain," Fatima laughed.

"Yes. Pigeons can remember over seven hundred visual patterns," Fiona added.

"I don't think humans could do that," Rowan admitted.

"Yes, but humans can write poetry," Fatima consoled.

"Some birds can also use elementary tools. Do you know that in the bushfires we have here in Australia, kites and falcons are known to carry small burning twigs and drop them to start new fires to flush their prey, a technique as you know, humans have use in war since biblical times. Perhaps we learnt this technique from these dinosaurs," Fiona explained further. She was remembering the scorched-earth policy often used by the military to destroy enemy assets.

"And the bird singing. That would interest you very much Rowan," Fatima said.

"As in our Indian movies where we have songs to attract a partner and strengthen the bond between partners," Rowan continued.

"I like to watch Indian dances," Fatima admitted.

"Bird songs and calls are most interesting aren't they?" Rowan said.

"And like us, birds have many local variations, or dialects, in different geographic areas," Fatima continued.

"Have you noted how birds have evolved in a way to turn selfish behaviour into communal cooperation, something we humans have tried to do for a long time? By feeding in different ways and in different parts of the tree or the water, these birds minimize the competition, so their individual selfish behaviour becomes a communal effort. Like long legged great egrets and blue herons feed in deeper water than the shorter legged ibises here in Australia," Fiona continued.

"I have seen pelicans, swans, great egrets, darters, cormorants on Lake Macquarie which is down the road from here," Fatima said.

"I really love their colourful feathers. Some Indian kingfishers are so beautiful. We have a beer in India named after them," Rowan continued.

"The colour serves many functions apart from species identification. It serves in courtship displays to attract a mate, like when we get dressed up for a social dance gathering," Fiona added.

"Like a bird lek?" Rowan asked.

"Exactly," Fiona was impressed Rowan knew about bird lekking.

"I saw a lekking display once. I was on a hiking trip in Sonkhaliya grasslands in Rajasthan in India. Great Indian bustards. There were about fifteen of them. It was exhilarating to watch," Rowan continued

"You are so lucky Rowan. I have never ever seen any lekking displays," Fiona admitted.

"Another reason for us to go to India to see lekking," Fatima said.

"In India we used to have some lekking displays among the boys trying to imitate *Elvis Presley's* dancing at social gatherings particularly when the girls watched."

"I'm sure you would have walked away with a sizeable amount of girls for your harem, Rowan," Fiona teased.

"I don't know about that. Indian girls are trained not to express their feelings as are also the men," Rowan said looking downwards. Obviously he was remembering something that had affected him deeply a long time ago. He remembered Mangala, a girl he liked at St. Xaviers College. She had beautiful black long hair. She had liked him too, he had deciphered. But it was meant not to happen. Grandma Felicity would never have allowed it.

"Shame," Fiona said.

"Birds are very promiscuous aren't they?" Fatima was confused in this aspect, it appeared.

"No, most birds are monogamous. Swans, petrels and parrots mate for life," Fiona responded.

"That's interesting," Rowan expressed his surprise.

"Only less than ten percent are promiscuous. But there are males who will mate with many females and there are females that will mate with many males. Many mating females allow for an increase in numbers, many mating males allow for an increase in variety," Fiona explained.

"Have you heard of our bowerbirds in Western Australia? The male birds actually decorate their nests with colourful objects to attract a female mate," Fatima continued.

"You know Fiona, I have often wondered why birds can't fly backwards. Is it because they know the world is round and they never need to go backwards?" Rowan asked.

"That may not be true Rowan. Humming birds can fly backwards," Fiona informed.

"Birds are an interesting subject. Aren't they? Thank you both. I have learned a lot today," Rowan concluded.

"You started it all Rowan. Thanks to you," Fatima finished.

And they were lost in meditation at the window for a while. The lapwing was gone and Rowan looked around to see if he could spot it. Fatima was wishing she could fly and what it would be like to fly and Fiona was feeling particularly knowledgeable in all birdy measures.

Almost as an afterthought Fiona mentioned, "It is interesting that we humans fight to kill, for territory defence. In birds it is mostly a highly ritualized behaviour. Injuries and deaths are relatively rare."

"Birds attempt to defend their territory with body postures, plumage displays, chase, and vocal noises. Actual fighting may occur only if these threats are ignored. Usually the objective is to hurt, not to kill so that the loser retreats away into another territory." Fatima explained.

Exactly at this moment as if planned, Faye entered the room and found them all looking out of the window.

"What's happening?' she inquired and hurried towards the window expecting some surprise.

"Nothing. We were just talking about birds," Fatima replied.

"Is Rowan a bird watcher?" Faye wanted to know.

"I have just been converted," Rowan smiled.

"Really. Fiona, did you tell him about all our loquacious parrots, parakeets, galahs, finches, kookaburras, emus and our mound builders in Western Australia?" Faye was keen to let Rowan know.

"No. We were just talking about birds in general," Fiona informed.

"We have a great variety of interesting birds here, Rowan. You will love them. We have birds that don't fly like penguins, we have gamebirds like pheasants, colourful parrots, hunting birds like falcons, water birds, seabirds and perching birds like finches," Faye continued providing her contribution to Rowan's impending interest.

"Yes it seems so," Rowan replied.

"Would you believe an American scientist, *Charles Sibley* showed Australia was the first home of the world's songbirds?" Faye continued.

"You are pulling my leg Faye after all the chirpers, screamers, screechers and yelpers I have encountered here," Rowan said.

"And we have snakes and spiders," Fatima joked.

"What? You love snakes and spiders Fatima?" Rowan asked.

"No, no. I just hate them," Fatima corrected.

"But we have to share Australia with them. If you leave them alone they will not interfere with you," Fiona pacified.

"Our budgerigars, you may know them as parakeets are very beautiful. The common ones are bright yellow and green, with a blue cheek and black scalloping on the wing feathers and a dark blue tail," Faye informed.

"Yes. I have seen those around," Rowan remembered. He had seen them around King Edward Park in his evening walking sessions from the hospital.

"They are usually found in the open plains and grasslands in large flocks. Some people have them as pets. They eat mainly grass seeds," Faye continued.

"The Australian magpie is one of the cleverest birds on earth. It has a beautiful song of extraordinary complexity. It can recognize and remember up to thirty different human faces," Fiona informed.

"Yes. The magpie is one of our most popular birds despite statistics showing that magpies stab the eyes of one or two people each year often causing permanent damage," Faye added.

"Generally Australian birds are more likely to eat sweet foods, lead long lives, live in complex societies, attack other birds and are intelligent and loud. I suppose the nature of our continent made them to be this way, to survive," Fiona added.

"Our finches are the greatest. My friend, Natalie's father has an aviary. He breeds them to sell. He has a beautiful collection of different varieties like Zebra, Gouldian and the like. If you want I can ask her if I can bring you along one day. Her father is a very nice man," Fatima said.

"I'd love to see them," Rowan replied.

"There is an interesting book by *Graham Pizzey* which lists all our Australian birds. I have a copy that you can borrow if you wish," Fatima offered.

"Yes, I would like to borrow that book from you tonight and also join you on your group excursions when I can," Rowan said. This is going to be interesting, he thought.

Having grown up in an urban city and with his busy schedule, there was never any time to be interested in birds although crows and pigeons were usually the ones rostered mainly to detract not attract attention, as the competition for food scraps was fierce between the feline, canine, bovine, avian and often human life in Bombay.

His reminiscing was cut short by Fatima, "What kind of birds do you have in India?"

Rowan would rather not have to answer the question as he was not prepared for an impressionable answer. Nevertheless he ventured, "India has a rich bird life. We have crows, sparrows, pigeons, koel. The peacock is our national bird. We also have parrots, bulbuls and mynas.

"What does a bulbul look like?"

There was a notable silence. Rowan was rolling his tongue in search of an answer.

Carmen, who was paying attention to the prevailing conversation shouted from the kitchen, "It is a nightingale."

"Why is it called a bulbul?" Fatima raised her voice in Carmen's direction.

"That's an Arabic name," Carmen shouted again.

"Are Indian mynas the same as Australian mynas?" Another query shifted from Fatima in Carmen's direction.

"Both are actually Indian mynas. I read that they were first brought into Australia to control caterpillars and other insects in market gardens around Melbourne," Carmen shouted.

Just then, James entered. "Hi everyone. What's happening? Where's the mum? Carmen where are you?"

Carmen who was in the kitchen appeared in the doorway, "I'm here. Just preparing some lunch."

"What's for lunch?" James asked.

"I overheard their conversation and I am ashamed to say that I have some tandoori chicken sandwiches."

"Ashamed, why?" James was puzzled.

And to a degree Fiona and Fatima were also puzzled.

But Faye understood what Carmen meant. She

realized that chickens were somehow not included in the current bird preservation fad.

"We have a lot of societies protecting various birds but chickens somehow are of no concern," Carmen explained.

"So are you going for chicken rights?" James joked.

"No. Just saying," Carmen responded.

"We all have double standards Carmen. We are angry with duck shooters but we will happily consume chicken from the supermarket. We cull feral cats to save endangered birds," Faye continued.

"Is there an answer?" Fatima asked.

"Ah, now I know where this conversation is coming from. In these matters we must not be consumed by others' opinions. Others may have vested interests such as a financial or some sort of self-promotion gain by exhibiting themselves as being different. After all, that's what it takes to be noticed. We must use our own logic and reason rather than rely on our emotions. Where does killing become murder? Where does eating become cannibalism? Most people are agreed that the line lies between humans and other species. Some draw the line at all animals excluding mice, insects or bacteria but will happily consume plant life. The very fact that life has always depended on a predator-prey race from the beginning of time should aid our thinking. The final choice is our own. And finally you need to decide if you like chicken tikka or Kentucky fried or Henny Penny or Red Rooster," James delivered his impromptu sermonette.

"I think we should have a pet budgie or maybe really a pair?" Fiona suggested. Everyone looked at her for a moment. No one wanted to consider this seriously.

"I want to recommend a book to you Fiona. It is called *Birdman of Alcatraz* by *Gaddis*," James said.

"You mean Thomas Gaddis. I read it in school. I found it a very moving and thought-provoking story of Robert Stroud," Rowan added.

"I read it a long time ago too. I remember it had a lot of thinking material for me too at the time," James added.

"Who is Robert Stroud?" was expected of Fatima.

"He was a notorious criminal who reared and sold birds from Leavenworth Penitentiary in the US and was later transferred to Alcatraz which is an island in the middle of San Francisco Bay," James answered.

"What Stroud accomplished in solitary confinement is much more than most free people do with far more resources and possibilities," Rowan said.

"What more did he do?" Faye asked.

"He learnt French and translated some of the French classics," Rowan informed.

"I was left with a couple of questions after reading the book. I remember thinking if he would have been better off, if he had instead been placed in a facility for the mentally challenged rather than a regular prison and was his mistake being too manipulative and constantly trying to challenge authority?" James asked.

"I remember Stroud is quoted in the epilogue of the book, 'I have demonstrated time and again that no man is or even can be defeated until he, himself, quits fighting' or something to that effect. That may answer your second question," Rowan remarked.

"Eventually I was left with the impression that Gaddis may have been a bit soft on Stroud in his book but nevertheless it is well worth reading," James looked toward Fiona.

"I think so too. A good read," Rowan echoed.

"I am going to get myself a copy," Carmen decided.

And tandoori chicken sandwiches were served and partaken delightedly by all.

A few days later, Carmen received two copies of the book presented to her, one from James and the other from Rowan. She gave one copy to Fiona.

30

A lone myna on the window sill was attempting to test the quadritone loudness tolerance of sentient life in the vicinity aided by other mates further away providing the intermittent chorus verses.

There was a scheduled hospital meeting for the consultants at the hospital from which James who had no appetite for hospital politics was abstaining, having provided his apologies. The evening sun was refusing obliteration on the horizon and was involved in its own tactics to achieve this goal, often attempting to hide behind passing clouds so the horizon could not find it.

Fatima entered the room where Carmen, Rowan and James were discussing the weather for tomorrow. She appeared quite perturbed as she sat down.

"You appear very upset my dear, what is the matter?" Carmen observed.

Fatima was as usual not very secretive of her inner plights and employed all her facial musculature to expose her inner self to those in the vicinity.

"I was reading an essay on beliefs and it was disturbing," Fatima opened up.

As if on cue Fiona and Faye wondered in together and took seats unaware of the prevailing conversation.

"What was disturbing Fatima?" Carmen wanted to know. She always had a soft corner for Fatima and her permanent curiosity and loved her for it.

"Well Carmen, it says the brain evolved to act but not necessarily to think. How can that be?" Fatima tried to explain her problem.

"Think of it this way Fatima. The brain absorbs information and creates or imagines still more of what it considers information and combines the two. In other words, it organises information for itself and is willing and often eager to explain to others what it has created. The brain along with its owner that is you, seems strongly inclined to believe what it explains. Together they predict events and initiate action or inaction. So really to act it has also to think," Carmen explained.

"Fatima, we humans have evolved from a long line of story tellers endowed by nature with a curious compulsion to account for everything, particularly the unaccountable. So it is the essence of our mind to find a causative agent for every event. The early Sumerians had five hundred and sixty gods to attribute events to. The mythology was then passed on from the Sumerians to the Arcadians to the Babylonians to the Asyrenians to the Eygptians. I hope I got that right," James paused to think and then continued, "So Egyptian religion and the associated how the universe began cosmogonies is the source of early Greek religion which next is taken up by the Romans. In each culture the names of the gods are selected appropriately to fit in with local mythic heroes. Marduk, Serapis, Isis, Zeus, Jupiter etcetera.

Ancient history shows that the victors usually succumbed to the religion of the conquered over a period of time. In these early times, polytheism prevailed. In later times, the conquerors forced their religion on the conquered. This occurred particularly in Christianity and Islam, often this being the only motive for the invasion. In these later times monotheism prevailed. Religion really requires stories and the stories occasionally overwhelm the facts," James explained, still feeling doubtful about the chronological sequences he had mentioned.

"So, really we have the same gods with different names in different cultures," Fatima summarised.

"It seems so," Faye understood similarly.

"Our brain aims for explanations and beliefs that may improve control over events and increase the odds of predictable outcomes. So the brain's job is to explain and assess and then to believe in its assessments and to try to govern action," Carmen continued.

"So the brain thinks as well as acts. Both? Think first act later," Fatima attempted to understand.

"The brain also imagines and believes things for which there is no hard evidence such as animals with human characteristics, hell, heaven, witches, angels and the like. Early people understood that gods could become human and humans could become gods," James added.

"So god to mortal and vice versa transition occurrences were accepted in earlier times?" Fatima queried.

Rowan, Fiona and Faye found it interesting and

were beginning to get their own antennas working.

"It seems religious ideas involve non-natural explanations just like our dreams," Faye observed.

"Exactly, because in both cases the left front cortex is involved. In our dreams, logic, reason, connection and causation, goes out of the window. This is something we never do in our waking life. Thus our dreams usually give us an impossible experience." Carmen explained from her knowledge of psychology. She remembered her lecturer, Mrs Percy Bhiwandiwalla at KC College fondly, who had said so. She also recollected Mrs Bhiwandiwalla always wore a blue sari. She could see Mrs Bhiwandiwalla now, in her own mind, standing at the minimally raised rostrum which contributed minimally to visually accessing her from her student seat.

Suddenly she heard her name mentioned and was transported back to the present.

"Like Carmen said, rituals often incorporate hallucinogenic drugs, trance, dance, meditation music and the like. All these rituals move us away from waking consciousness and provide non-natural, dreamlike experience guided by the left cortex," James explained further.

"And reinforce the religious impulse," Rowan was beginning to bend in his beliefs having seen the logic.

"So on some level, we are hard-wired, or at least strongly predisposed to believe things we cannot prove." Fiona surmised.

"That's what we need to fight and correct in ourselves," James added.

"Let me summarise this slowly. Correct me if I am

wrong. So eventually beliefs are formed from a variety of subjective, personal, emotional, and psychological reasons in the light of the facts provided to us through the filters of our hunches, biases, and prejudices created by family, friends, colleagues, culture, and society at large," Rowan ventured.

"Very beautifully put Rowan," Fiona complimented him. Carmen looked proudly at Rowan.

"And then after forming our beliefs as you suggest Rowan, we then defend, justify, and rationalise them with a host of intellectual reasons, cogent arguments, and rational explanations. Our perceptions about reality are dependent on the beliefs that we hold about it. The human mind thus becomes essentially a belief machine," James added.

"Religious faith is not amenable to reason and when we make people choose between faith and reason, some will choose faith and then go on to defend it and their choice by rejecting reason and evidence," Fiona added.

"I would have thought that as the level of education increases, superstitious beliefs would decrease," Fatima said.

"No, I have seen some very smart people who believe bizarre things. I think they don't want to be considered stupid at this stage of their life and so they will defend the beliefs they arrived at for non-smart reasons earlier. And when that does not work they will even resort to abusive language or violence if needed," Faye added.

Carmen was listening intently to the non-emotional argumentation. She had more thinking and rethinking to do. Up that slope again.

"Take the Gospels for example," James started, "They were written about seventy five years later, not by eyewitnesses but by Greek speaking non Palestines who loved to tell a good story. The first one was Matthew. He never mentions that Mary was a virgin. This mention would really have provided a great substance for his story. The next in line was Mark who merely copies Mathew and moulds the story to adhere with what the scriptures say, by making Mary a virgin. Luke copies further and adds the annunciation. But the best of the fiction writing ever produced is provided by John in his accounts of the miracles. If there were really any miracles don't you think the previous authors would have mentioned them? Would it not have helped their own story immensely? "

Within themselves both Carmen and now Rowan realised they had a lot of thinking to do on that front. They had logical thinking to contend with as well as the spiritual deceit they had been subjected to by the Christian clergy in Byculla. Carmen had already been on the other side before with James. She remembered she had felt so much lighter in those days without all the Christian bandages. She could do it easily again, now that her position with James and the girls was quite secure. Rowan thought he would have problems, but then, he himself could think and reason well. Essentially he adored James and he knew that James would had explored all his subject topics very thoroughly. Such was the nature of James.

"I think I will dance" Fiona jumped up suddenly and, "Rowan will you join me?"

"Of course," Rowan obliged. Rock and roll without audible music it was.

"I will go and listen to some music," Faye decided and left the room.

"And I will meditate," Fatima laughed.

"And I will have some wine," James added, "Carmen will you join me?"

"Yes, most definitely. I need some after all that."

James got up and fetched two glasses of wine. He offered one to Carmen, "That was an interesting conversation. Thank you Carmen."

"Not me. Fatima really started it," Carmen replied.

"I love you all. Om Om Om," Fatima mouthed loudly.

"Eventually faith is dependent only on the trusting of a source. Isn't it? Reason is dependent on evidence and logic, it is learned," James was now on fire.

"I can't argue with that," Carmen admitted.

"In my opinion if there is only one theory on a subject and it has lasted for a long time, we should accept it until it is proved wrong, like for example the theory of gravity. But if there two theories on a subject contradicting each other, then one may be true and the other is definitely wrong because both can't be true and particularly if they contradict each other and if there are three or more than they are all wrong like all the various religions we have," James added.

Carmen looked at James and wrinkled her forehead. James has not succumbed in his views of religion and is sounder than ever. She thought 'I do love you James in spite of'.

Faye returned. It was obvious she had a fresh problem on her mind now.

"I have been thinking about the ten commandments. The Abrahamic God appears to be a narcissist and is more concerned about his own feelings that our wellbeing. The majority of his commandments are not about morality, but about worshipping him," Faye was clearly upset.

"Yes that has occurred to me before, but I have always put it under the carpet," Fiona replied. She and Rowan stopped dancing.

"Someone has to be the devil's advocate or rather god's advocate in this matter. Any volunteers? What about you James?" Rowan provoked.

"Over my not yet dead body," James laughed.

"The first four commandments all refer to 'the lord thy god' who really appears vain, and like most dictators, must resort to threats, rather than any intellectual persuasion, to promote a point of view. They are so petty and reflect a very insecure god," Faye continued.

"As usual we must first consider if the event is even likely to have happened. For example take the matter of Jesus. We are told he rose from his tomb after the stone was shifted and whilst the guarding soldiers were sleeping. Jesus was crucified as a criminal according to Roman law. The worst punishment in Roman law was crucifixion. The Romans buried their criminals in mass graves. And these are historical facts. When a fact is altered to suit a narrator's point of view, the result is fiction. It is not possible that he was allocated a separate tomb particularly if the jury comprised mainly of Jews. If someone rises from a mass grave how do we know it is Jesus? So you have to invent a separate tomb for the story to hang.

Similarly on Mount Sinai which is two thousand, two hundred and eighty five metres high, first we must consider if the event actually took place. Consider an almost eighty year old man climbing it alone. He was gone for forty days without food and water. And god appears to him only when he is alone! Today we know such physical depletions can cause hallucinations!"

"Yes, its most likely it never ever happened and is just a story," Fatima said.

"Nevertheless, Commandments six through nine— thou shalt not kill, commit adultery, steal or bear false witness are good, but they need a big revision in today circumstances. There are no commandments against slavery, bias, rape or incest or child molestation," Faye continued.

"These things were not expected to happen in god's great plan for humanity," James joked.

"No that was not god's fault. It was the serpent or Eve again at fault. The serpent must have slipped her another apple," Rowan decided to join in.

"The tenth commandment, does not allow the desire of thy neighbour's wife, neither shalt thou covet thy neighbour's house, his field etcetera which really treats women as inanimate property. One thing we can be sure of is that god can't be a woman." Fiona said.

"Even coveting is a sin, would you believe it?" Fatima observed.

"And if god is a man then all men who love god are

poofs," Faye was clearly upset.

"Many of the gods, Jupiter, Zeus including the Holy Ghost would lose on coveting. Coveting and getting poor Joseph's wife pregnant," James mentioned.

"Little in Christianity is original. Most smart children could come up with a much superior list of commandments quite easily," Fatima deciphered.

"I agree there is a serious need to change the commandments. But dogma and tradition will always prevail in the church. There is only one commandment in my book. Thou shall not engage in human trafficking whether physical or mental," Rowan volunteered after giving serious consideration to the matter within himself, as to whether he should participate fully in this discourse or not. He was beginning to realise that common sense and reason must always prevail in all matters and he had been a sucker too long. He thought that faith is for those unable to think and for those who are very comfortable with cognitive dissonance demanding reason in all matters outside religion. Really scientists who profess faith must be the ones who can compartmentalise two incompatible worldviews in their heads.

"The Church has its own nonnegotiable foundation which cannot be rejected as the entire institution will collapse if it moves. Don't forget papal infallibility and the general apathy of thinking Christians of attempting to move a papal mountain," James continued.

"Even the Muslim Koran has similar commandments. Of interest is, 'If anyone has killed one person it is as if he had killed the whole of mankind. The believers are those who do not call upon another god alongside Allah or kill the soul which Allah has made sacred. The killer is not a believer while he is killing," Rowan informed.

"I think we have defined the real meaning of bullshit today," James concluded." Can I top your glass again Carmen. What about you Rowan, Fiona, Faye, Fatima any for you?"

"Yes we all need some, I think," Fiona spoke.

"Not for me. I am on call" Rowan said.

"I will have some and also Rowan's share," Fatima joked.

"In all this it is important to always be able to think for yourself, remembering to know that there are a number of thinking fallacies and biases we all have that interfere with our ability to reason clearly and rationally," James spoke as he was pouring the wine.

"What are they?" Fiona wanted to know.

" Always proportion your belief to the evidence available, don't be fooled by fantastic stories," James began.

"In that regard a common way of being fooled is by overestimating the power of anecdotes or stories. Our tendency is to believe whatever we hear and anecdotes can be powerful belief fuel," Fiona had realised.

"Anecdotes are not data," Rowan was hard in the conversation now. Carmen was observing him with pride. He was beginning to escape what she had been forced into from childhood. Hopefully his grandmother, Felicity was not watching him from above.

"Another common mistake in our thinking is that if we cannot explain something, it must be inexplicable and, therefore, a true mystery of god. Even reasonable people sometimes think that if the experts cannot explain something, it must be inexplicable. There are many genuine unsolved mysteries in the universe, and it is always acceptable to express our lack of understanding which in time will be amenable to a solution. After all we have been on this earth for only two hundred thousand years and most of the time we could not or were not allowed to think for ourselves," James continued.

"The problem is that all of us find it more comforting to have certainty than to live with unsolved or unexplained mysteries," Rowan said.

"Rain gods provide certainty in stormy weather for sailors maybe," Fatima said.

"In the world of the gods, coincidences are often seen as deeply significant," James added. Such topics really got James fired and he came alive having given them much prior significant consideration, both in his extensive reading and his thinking.

Carmen was feeling left out although she agreed in all that was said. She now began, "When dealing with events that seem unusual, we must ask how likely is such a thing to occur given all the relevant factors?"

"That's a very important consideration Carmen. Thank you," James complimented her after noticing she had been mostly silent thus far.

"The Bermuda Triangle mystery provides an interesting example. Those who believe that there is something supernatural at work don't know the baseline rate of accidents for the area. Far more shipping lanes run through the Bermuda Triangle than the surrounding areas. Accidents and disappearances are more likely to happen in that area. Ironically, the accident rate is actually lower in the Bermuda Triangle than in surrounding areas," Carmen was definitely livening up to the discussion.

"We should look for probable worldly explanations before turning to otherworldly ones. Before we say that something is out of this world, we should first make sure that it is not in this world," Rowan continued.

"Some people think that if you cannot disprove a claim, it must be true. But belief must come from positive evidence in support of a claim, not lack of evidence for or against a claim. Also discrediting one position does not force the acceptance of the other," James continued. There was no stopping him now. The wine was being ignored.

"Many times we find ourselves trapped in circular reasoning. Christianity is filled with repetitions such as, 'Is there a God? Yes. How do you know? Because the Bible says so. How do you know the Bible is correct? Because it was inspired by God.'In other words, God is… because God is." James continued.

"Some people say that it would be an evil world without religion," Fiona was being an unofficial god's advocate.

"What do you think?" James asked.

"How much more than it is now, with all the religions we have, Fiona?" Rowan asked.

"Religion keeps the already good people, good. It does not make the bad people good. Several Christian popes are the very best testimony to this fact," Fatima added.

"An excellent observation Fatima," James complimented her.

"Can we have the wine now?" Fatima asked. The throats were getting thirsty.

"Sorry folks" James apologised and went to pouring the wine again.

It had been an interesting conversation, Carmen thought. She would have to go to her own drawing board again!

Rowan reminded himself again about how lucky he was that James was his biological father. He really had no real heavenly father as he had until recently believed! Thank you James!

Rowan excused himself and took himself off to bed.

The wine was consumed slowly with everyone lost in private thoughts until it was time to go to bed. It had been a very fruitful discussion.

"Just leave the glasses in the sink. I will attend to them tomorrow," were Carmen's last words before going to bed. She was physically and mentally tired and hoped James was too.

31

The days passed uneventfully and one evening after partaking of a tasty Indian dinner contributed to by the efforts of Carmen and the three girls, the family settled in the lounge room for an after dinner hexalogue. The remnant food odours emanating from the kitchen, possibly unaware of the phenomenon of smell adaptation were determined to make their presence felt irrespective. The chandelier sprinkled its photo manipulating effects around confusing the deep red coloured sofas which were delighting in accommodating it's occupants. The moon had decided to take the night off and the stars alone were deployed to provide the entertainment for the poetic and religious minds.

Both James and Rowan were on call for the hospital. Being on call was generally a stressor, not for the complexity of cases encountered but just for the fact that one could not relax. Generally Rowan had observed that if one attempted to relax, the number of calls would increase. If one remained tense, there were usually no calls. The obvious option then was to remain tense and pretentiously relaxed.

Fatima as usual gave vent to her curiosity, which characteristic about her, actually also pleased James very much. He was grateful for her discourses. She always created an excellent and informative conversation in the family and always got everyone interested, thinking and contributing. It was reminiscent of his own childhood.

"Dad, I read today that platypuses have a duck bill, a beaver tail and an otter body and fur. When we saw it at the zoo last time, it did not occur to me that it was really a hodgepodge."

"I had a penfriend in Canada who told me about beaver tails but that was a pastry apparently," Rowan reminisced rolling his tongue. By this stage he had given up in attempting to control his tongue. He thought that if James had not succeeded by now, his own chances were minimal.

"It is an interesting curiosity. Isn't it? Almost oneiric. It is one of the great marvels of evolution we still have only here in Australia. All our big animals disappeared with the human occupation of our continent," Fiona joined in.

"Evolution is very interesting. It is a simple natural selection to suit the prevailing circumstances. The platypus was left behind when Australia separated from Pangea as Rowan mentioned and it really required no real reason for further adaptation as it had no natural predators here," Faye commented.

"The platypus is the only remaining descendant of an ancestor that diverged from all the other mammals about one hundred and fifty million years ago," James added.

"Yes. The way natural selection moulds a species depends on very unpredictable changes in the climate and sometimes on random physical events such as meteor strikes or volcanic eruptions and on which species happens to be lucky enough to survive a mass extinction," Rowan added, rolling his tongue at his every intended punctuation and went on further, "and on the occurrence of rare and random beneficial mutations."

To him this topic was intriguingly interesting and was not to be taken lightly. He had read widely about it and in fact had spent many an hour thinking about it sometime ago. His mind was often kept busy by auto-argumentation and this topic was often a big contender. He was grateful to Fatima for bringing it up. He would get to know everyone's views and particularly James', which he very much looked forward to. Australia with all its varied collection of mammals was a great support for evolution. He only hoped the phone would not ring this evening.

"Evolution is really very unpredictable isn't it? We don't know exactly how the environment will change or what mutations will occur," Fiona reiterated.

"Also predators can force it's own prey to evolve and prey can force it's own predators to evolve for survival," Fatima said. She was obviously thinking of the cheetah and the gazelle competition for survival in the African savannah.

"Exactly. Reproductive output is the currency of natural selection and reproduction is helped sometimes by evolution's removal of features that aren't useful. It seems complexity is not always favoured by natural selection. Nature constantly makes new variants, mostly inferior, a few superior, and all of these variants must pass through the filter of natural selection. Natural selection can preserve such innovations, but it cannot create them. Given enough time, this explains all of the variations we have today," James explained with his own version of tongue rolls.

"Actually there are five important evolutionary mechanisms," Rowan was on fire now and recruited his fingers out to support and with his tongue rolling, "let me see - mutation, genetic drift, gene flow, non-random mating, and natural selection." He put his fingers away and continued further, "Genetic drift is simply the random changes in the proportion of genes caused by reproduction. If some genes make no difference to the number of offspring, the proportion of those genes in a population would simply fluctuate at random. This really does not matter to adaptation. But natural selection does produce adaptation. This gives an organism a reproductive advantage in its current circumstances as Faye mentioned."

It helped that he had considered evolution in depth some time ago particularly when he used to go on those long walks by himself after dinner on the Newcastle foreshore and he was all set for today's conversation. Bring it on!

"So natural selection only selects what is already there," Fatima summarised.

"Exactly," James replied.

"It's amazing how any god can be so wasteful rejecting the nonadapters and letting them die," Faye added.

"Good point Faye. Actually the innovations come from old existing things to make the new. Like building a new kind of car from old car parts. Many mutations neither harm nor help when they first occur, "James continued.

"Mutations relating to brain function may create slight alterations in proteins in turn, shaping differences in behaviour for adaptation. Our minds can also evolve to cope with environmental variability," Carmen offered. She was homing for evolutionary psychology.

"Individuals are naturally selected to behave in their own reproductive interests and the fate of the species as a whole is not relevant to any individual's reproductive decisions," James continued further.

"I know that two siblings share roughly fifty per cent of their genes from a common ancestor parent, while two cousins share twelve and a half per cent, which they inherit from a grandparent," Faye added attempting to bring in what she had learnt from her her school yard conversations.

"Human and chimpanzee lineages separated around five million years ago," Rowan contributed to the hexalogue at this stage.

"Our genus appeared two and half million years ago. The Neanderthals appeared in Europe in the Ice Age. *Homo sapiens* where we belong came from Africa. The oldest human remains in Australia were found at Lake Mungo in south-west New South Wales. This site has been occupied by Aboriginal people for at least forty seven thousand years ago to the present," James continued mainly for Fatima's benefit.

"We are most closely related by DNA to pygmy

chimpanzees and gorillas. We share about ninety-eight per cent of our DNA with them," Rowan offered.

"And yet we shut them up in zoos and conduct experiments on them?" Faye was demonstrating her activist tendencies.

"Hitler did that to the Jews and the white Americans did that to the black Americans. No point in chasing that path today Faye. 'Let bygones be bygones' as mum always says to me," Rowan replied as Carmen smiled.

James understood what Carmen had meant. He only just wished he himself had done things differently in his own life sometimes.

Carmen seemed unperturbed, "Just continuing what I mentioned before, behaviours are adaptations produced by the process of natural selection. Much of our behaviour is not in keeping with today's age because we are stuck with a Stone Age mindset in a modern environment. And so we have problems like anxiety and depression which behaviours that were necessary in the Stone Age for survival," Carmen added.

"Really. How did anxiety and depression help at that time mother?" Rowan was keen to know as were the others.

"Well, fear and anxiety causes us to avoid danger doesn't it? And depression causes us to stay away at home and gives us time to recover," Carmen explained.

"Yes I see it now. Very interesting," Rowan replied.

"Thanks Carmen. That is interesting," Faye echoed.

"Our environment has never been stable at any time in the Earth's history and any species that had rigid mechanisms would definitely never survive," James said.

"It seems natural selection is not random but mutation is random," Fatima said. She was finding all this very interesting and challenging.

"Exactly, that hits the nail on it's head Fatima," James complimented her understanding.

"Evolution seems just like a form of descent with some modification. Its almost like music to me. People come up with different songs. Depending on the prevailing tastes, some survive and some don't make it," Faye said. She had remembered the recent discourse on music.

"Good analogy Faye," James complimented her.

"That's a nice observation Faye. The new song has most of the characteristics of the last successful song with a little tweak," Carmen contributed.

"That's why we rock and rolled from jazz as Rowan said," Fatima continued.

"*Charles Darwin* put everything on a sound scientific footing," James added.

"He was not even aware that he had received the Nobel Prize at the time that it was actually happening, as his son's funeral was taking place at the same time. Very sad," Rowan remembered.

With that information the participants were immersed in a round of melancholy and silence prevailed for a little while. Even great men have some tragedy in their lives James was reminded.

"The greatest evidence we have for evolution is

fossils and fossil layers, the similarities among organisms today, similarities in DNA, and similarities of the stages the embryo goes through," Rowan began again.

"Will evolution ever stop?" Fatima had to ask.

"The only way to truly stop any biological organism from evolving is its extinction.

"Evolution can be slowed by reducing and keeping population size to a small number of individuals. This will lead to a loss of most genetic variation through genetic drift and minimize the input of new mutations into the population," Rowan had worked this out in his private monologues. He had often thought about the effects of enforced birth control in India.

"Are we still evolving?" Fatima inquired after a while.

"Yes we are. All organisms are dynamic and moving on with evolution. As you can see in our own family, the mixing of human populations is already well underway and such mixing will continue to homogenize our species. Rowan is ahead of us already," James said.

Rowan felt elated briefly. Me, ahead of James? Not possible he thought.

"Fatima, this is another reason for us to visit India. We can find an Indian partner and take a step ahead in evolution for our children," Fiona said gleefully.

Rowan smiled. He had thought of James' statement. He had a different opinion to offer, "James, I really do not think we are evolving biologically anymore. We have taken control of most of our threats. We do not have any predators. In fact we are the only real predators on this earth. I think human evolution has stopped because humans now adapt to their environment via cultural evolution and not biological evolution"

"I see your point but I think both kinds of evolution are proceeding side by side. What you say fits in nicely with the *Niche construction theory* if you have heard of it," James said.

"No. What's that?" Rowan was interested

"Adaptation does not look like a one way process anymore. Organisms do not respond entirely to the environment only. Organisms can make problems for themselves, as well as solving problems set by the environment. Also niche-constructing activities do not have to be genetically based. Learning, and other forms of experience, may lead to animal niche construction. In humans, we are prodded on by culture," James explained.

"Talking about predators, how did we get here?" Faye asked.

"Yes, we are not very big nor can we run very fast," Fiona added.

"No. but we have guns and gun powder," Rowan explained.

"So which way and where do you think we are now going dad?" Faye asked.

"We have two qualities that may destroy us all. It is our tendency to kill each other and to destroy the environment. If we overcome these tendencies, then it is possible that we will probably have a civilization on Mars or the Moon, or who knows maybe even another planet beyond the solar system. We have discovered billions and billions of planets outside our own solar system. There are forty billion Earth-like planets in our own galaxy alone."

"Yes we may need to de-evolve very heavily for that. Perhaps give up our dependency on oxygen and water. Perhaps learn to photosythesise, learn to hibernate, learn to fly," Rowan laughed.

The conversation was now getting too probabilistic but somehow everyone seemed very interested.

"Could there be life out there?" Carmen wanted to know.

"I think so. But they are very likely not to be in the right step with us. They are either very far advanced or very far behind. So communicating with them may not be possible, it seems to me," James replied attempting to control his tongue rolling. He had read that somewhere before. Maybe it was *Carl Segan* he thought.

"They could be a non carbon, non water based creature," Rowan had to offer rolling his tongue.

"Yes. In which case they can't really be life as we see it," Fiona said.

"So we will not be able to identify them even if we see, hear or feel them," Carmen worked out.

"Yes they might have different sensors," Rowan said.

"So we could never become universal predators could we?" Fatima asked.

"Seems so. But then, I have been wrong before," James admitted.

"Considering we have a tendency to kill each other do you think life out there has already killed itself so that is why we have had no visitors?" Fiona asked.

"That is a very distinct possibility Fiona. Good observation," James said.

"Do you think humans can breed with any other animals?" Fatima queried next.

"Interesting thought Fatima," Faye was impressed.

"Most unlikely. Human DNA has become so different from that of other animals that interbreeding would likely be almost impossible. But please don't quote me on that. There's probably another *Victor Frankenstein* somewhere out there doing some unfunded research on that. Human nature has always been curious in this regard," Rowan replied.

"On a similar note do you think in the distant future, humans could become immortal?" Fiona asked.

"Good question Fiona. Wouldn't you like that? I don't know," James replied.

"I don't think living forever would be a good idea," Carmen intervened.

"Before male female sexes came in there was no death. Organisms continued forever just by dividing," Rowan offered.

"Yes. Interesting thinking Rowan," James commented. This thought had also occurred to him before somewhere, exactly where he could not remember now. James wondered how much more Rowan's thinking may also be akin his own.

"There is a type of jelly fish that can go back in its own lifecycle," Rowan informed.

"It seems we are now drifting rudderless into fantasies. But it is good. Yesterday's fantasies are today's facts," James said.

"Yes. We need hard statistics to deal with some of these probabilities. A kind of statistics we really don't have," Rowan finished.

"Thank god," Fiona uttered.

"What god? That too we don't have. I think we should go to bed now before our phones get woken up," James laughed.

"I think so," Carmen added. She only hoped James was not sexually aroused for more bedtime probabilities. And indeed he was not as she later found out.

"That was a very interesting conversation. I really enjoyed that. Thank you, everyone," Rowan finished.

The goodnight chorus was exchanged before everyone made their way out for their belated appointment with sleep.

32

The family was nestled in the lounge room, each engrossed in their own thoughts for the moment and James was perusing the local newspaper. Rowan was engrossed in a novel about the *Moulin Rouge* cabaret in Paris and *Henri de Toulouse-Lautrec*. Carmen was reading her copy of *Birdman of Alcatraz*. It was a quiet pleasant evening.

"Dad we should go for a picnic tomorrow if you and Rowan are not on call," Faye started.

Rowan put his book down and looked at James for a clue about his response.

"We are not on call," Rowan informed.

"That is a very good idea Faye. How do you feel Carmen?" James looked at Carmen.

"That's fine. I can prepare the food," Carmen declared.

"Let's go to Monkey Face Lookout in the Watagans. We have not been there for a long while," Fiona added.

James remembered that the last time they had been there was in his good times with Freida and the girls. Why did Fiona suggest the Watagans? Had she some issues to settle there? Would he be able to handle his own emotions? But by now James had learnt to prefer the reality of the present to the guilt of the past or the anxiety of the future.

"Okay that's fine," James agreed.

"That would be very nice," Fatima was joyed and attempted her usual happiness demonstration jig.

"Is that final? We can go then?" Faye asked again.

"Done Faye. Thanks for the suggestion. I am sure Carmen and Rowan will like the Watergans," James confirmed.

"How far is it?" Rowan asked rolling his tongue. He wanted to know.

"About an hour from here. We will take the Land Rover," James answered.

They hit the sack early and woke up early next morning. They were all wearing jeans and tropical coloured tops covered their upper torsos.

"We can easily find each other in the crowd with all these colours," Fatima observed.

"This is like being in India without the saris. In India we just love colours," Carmen said.

"Yes we look like a bunch of tropical birds," James joked.

"Me peacock you rainbow lorikeet," Fatima laughed pointing to Rowan.

"No, me pitta bird," Rowan said.

"What is a pitta bird?" Fiona asked.

"The Indian Pitta bird has nine colours and is called Nourang which means nine colours in Hindi," Rowan explained.

"That's interesting. What colours does it have?" Fiona asked.

"If I can remember correctly, brown, black, white, turquoise blue, buff, orange-red, pink, cerulean blue and green. Did I get nine?" Rowan asked rolling his tongue.

"Yes you did. I was counting," Fatima said.

"The most interesting birds are in South America. I would like to go there someday just to see the birds," Fiona admitted.

"I will come with you," Faye joined in.

"Me too. Dad can we go?" Fatima inquired.

"Someday," James offered.

"Don't forget your binoculars and cameras," Fiona reminded everyone.

The drive in the Land Rover was adventurously bumpy. James' lower back was attention demandingly, painful. He had some lower back pain for some time now which he attributed to his long operating hour sessions often with dysergonomic postures.

The sun was just embarking on its daily schedule. A mild wind was finding its path ushering the leaves out of its way and disembarking its cargo of wombat urine smell. The Monkey Face lookout views across the Martinsville Valley were brilliant. James thought that the aerial perspective with the bluish hued mountains would have *Tom Roberts* very busied with his oil paints. Some black cockatoos positioned themselves to be photographed much to Rowan's delight.

The girls found a beautiful quasi-bucolic spot. James was pleased to note that there were no overwhelming barbecuing beer logged men with their female acquisita and the usual accompanying paraphernalia of distressed children attempting conversation with the strangers in the vicinity.

James passed the cold beers around and they drank directly from the bottles.

"Beautiful sky. I love those clouds," Fatima was gazing upwards.

"Those are cumulus clouds. With the blue skies around, our weather today is assured," James observed.

"Would you like to eat something? I made some samosas and tandoori chicken pieces," Carmen interrupted.

"We're okay for the moment I think. Thank you Carmen," James replied.

"Just asking," Carmen responded.

"Does anyone know anything about clouds?" Fatima asked.

"I learned about clouds in school. Basically there are stratus clouds which are flat, cumulus clouds which are puffy and nimbus clouds which bear rain. And then you decide how high they are. The highest clouds have the prefix cirro. So a cirrostratus cloud would be a very high level flat cloud. These look like a frosted window pane. Mid-level clouds have the prefix of alto in front of them. The lowest level clouds don't have a prefix in them," Fiona volunteered as her attempt at information.

"So Fiona, our clouds today are cumulus clouds. No prefix," Fatima continued still looking upwards.

"Yes, that's right."

"What about nimbus clouds?" Carmen wanted to know.

"Nimbostratus is a routine rain bearing cloud whereas a cumulonimbus means impending thunderstorms"

"Is that all there is to know?" Fatima asked.

"No Fatima. Lots and lots more depending on the winds. That is why the weather bloke gets it wrong most of the time," Fiona explained.

"It is amazing that our ancestors looked at the clouds and saw their mysteries, myths, magic, miracles all there. We were so gullible then," Faye added.

James was pleased within himself. He had always believed in cautious curiosity. All his children were curious and willing to share their knowledge. He had often seen Rowan involved with the junior residents and the time and trouble he took in explaining to them.

He imagined how Rowan might have worked those long hours in Bombay, in his training days. He remembered the times in his own student days when senior doctors used intimidation to explain something implying that one must be dense not to get it and making one feel incapable of understanding it and leaving one the only option of committing it to memory. He remembered these academic bullies. He had learnt that with them no questions must be asked and he had resolved he would never be the same himself. His thoughts were interrupted when Carmen continued with the flavour of the current conversation.

"In Bombay we have four seasons, summer, winter, monsoon and the withdrawal season. December to February is the winter season, March to May is summer, June to September is monsoon season which seems like forever while October to December is the withdrawal season," Carmen informed.

"Here, we have summer from December to the end of February which is really the dry season, autumn from March to May which is the rainy season, winter from June to August, and spring from September to November which is the cyclone season," Faye provided the local information.

"You will have to forget Indian weather and get used to our weather now Carmen," James smiled.

"Indeed. I love the hot days," Carmen admitted.

"Yeah, I love the hot dry weather too. In Bombay it is humid," Rowan agreed.

"Time for some food now," Carmen saw her opportunity to dispose of some of her culinaries.

Carmen fetched the *samosas and tandoori chicken* and soft drinks and put them on in the picnic mat that Fiona and Rowan had spread. The ground wind was mild having spent it's major energy doing battle with the taller vegetation along the way.

The flies saw Carmen's unintended invitation as risky but a worth it enterprise. They had never alighted on samosas or tandoori chicken before and their chances of visiting India to partake of some such in their lifetime were marginal. So it had to be a do or die mission. Rowan having equipped himself with a fly swatter was determined to make it an impossible mission for them. Nevertheless, however hard he tried, he was not totally successful in providing a non-natural death to the flies, often having to apologise to the human recipients of his swatting efforts particularly Fiona. The flies were humiliating him massively in his efforts!

He thought about how any intelligent being could have ever made flies. The origin of life now made way into his thoughts. He wanted to know what the others had to say, "I wonder how life began on our planet?"

The girls who were usurped in Carmen's food dispensing efforts looked at Rowan. An interesting topic they all thought.

James was occupied in depriving a chicken drumette of the last of its fleshy component, ventured first, "Evidence locked in the earth's most ancient rocks suggests that by about 3.8 billion years ago, tiny bacteria had emerged"

"Yes but I mean before that," Rowan pointed out.

"I'm getting there. Life probably arose as a sequence of steps, first with the synthesis of simple organic molecules. Then the combination of these into larger macromolecules possibly occurred in a variety of different environments adding diversity to the molecular structure. Eventually, a self-replicating collection of macromolecules emerged of an increasing complexity and mutability through the process of natural selection, driven by competition for limited raw materials. And that's the beginning of evolution."

"Do we have any evidence for these steps?" Rowan inquired.

"Apart from logical thinking, no. Most of that history would be lost, because when later cells emerged, they would quickly consume virtually all traces of the earlier stages of chemical evolution for food."

At this stage Carmen's patience was beginning to run out a bit with Rowan's query which was introducing competition for her food disposal attempts, "You better eat some food now Rowan," she admonished.

"Wait mum. James, it must have arisen from chemical reactions among the oceans, the atmosphere, and rocks right?"

"Possibly the ocean," James replied.

"Okay, problem solved. Time for some food Rowan," Carmen started again.

Rowan saw there was no way out of Carmen's persistence. He remembered Carmen's firm determinations in forcing food on him even as a child. He gave in and picked up the nearest chicken morsel.

"It's a beautiful view of the valley here," Fatima said.

"What valley is that?" Rowan asked

"Martinsville valley," Fatima answered.

"Martinsville," Rowan repeated slowly.

"The view is magnificent because the pollution and moisture in the air is low here," James explained.

"Breathe as deep as you can for as long as you can. You may be able to pay your clean air mortgage sooner," Faye demonstrated with a few breaths that almost unbalanced her.

"Unfortunately not, my debt from the city is too high," Fiona replied.

As the food was finding its ultimate destination slowly and the flies were having a respite from Rowan's interference with their livelihood, Rowan's mind was not resting. Okay he thought life began, but how did it proceed? Did it get more complex just through chemistry or genetics? Perhaps James had read about it, he thought. Should he ask? And risk Carmen's harassing again? He decided not. Maybe another time.

Meanwhile Fatima was amassing her own questions, "So Fiona what affects the weather that we see?"

"That is a very big question but I will try."

"I want to know Fiona. I mean why do we have different types of weather?" Fatima persisted.

"This is almost a lecture Fatima. Do you still want to know?"

Carmen realised she was losing and decided to support Fatima's curiosity.

"I do too, Fiona. We are all ears," Carmen replicated Fatima's request.

"To understand that first we must know about air masses and the interactions between them. This is particularly important in the temperate zones where transitions between warm and cold air masses create zones of precipitation called fronts," Fiona started.

"So what exactly is an air mass?" Fatima asked.

"Its a body or a mass of air that has uniform temperature, pressure, and humidity throughout. Such air masses can stretch across hundreds of miles or more. Air masses originating over land are called continental and are dry, while air masses that form over water are called maritime and are moist. The boundaries between the air masses are called fronts."

"Why are they called fronts?" Carmen asked.

"Perhaps the term was borrowed from World War I where the dividing lines between battling armies were called fronts," James guessed.

"But weather fronts have existed before World War I," Rowan was not convinced.

"Yes, but weather fronts were perhaps not understood before," James added.

"Dad do you mind? Fiona please continue," Fatima did not like interferences. She usually listened intently and hated any distractions.

"Sorry," James apologised. He was usually aware of Fatima's preferences.

"Fronts are named after the type of air mass that is about to overtake another one.

So a cold front occurs when a cold air mass overtakes or displaces warm air, and a warm front occurs when a warm air mass displaces a cold air mass," Fiona continued. What she had learnt in school during dear Miss Dreary's talks was finally coming to be useful. And once Fiona started to talk about something she knew well, nothing including rain and thunderstorms could stop her.

"The signs of an approaching front are very distinctive, with wind and cloud patterns appearing in advance of the front. Warm fronts usually bring rain and cold fronts bring thunderstorms. Wind patterns are clockwise in the northern hemisphere and counter clockwise in the southern hemisphere," Fiona continued.

"Why?" Fatima asked.

"That's the Coriolis effect. Due to the Earth's rotation on its axis, the circulating air is deflected toward the right in the Northern Hemisphere and toward the left in the Southern Hemisphere, "James explained.

"The effect is zero at the equator and maximum at the poles. That is why there are no cyclones around the equator," Rowan helped.

"When the wind speed exceeds one hundred and twenty kilometres per hour, the cyclones are classified as either a hurricane or a typhoon, depending on where they form. In the Atlantic Ocean, they're called hurricanes, while in the Pacific, they're called typhoons. And that's all I know about weather. If you want to know more you, you will have to read it yourself Fatima," Fiona concluded.

"That was very good Fiona. After all that talking, more chicken for you?" Carmen asked.

"No thanks Carmen. I have had enough," Fiona replied.

"Thank you for that Fiona," Fatima looked toward Fiona.

"I remember the Coriolis effect being explained as throwing a ball to someone on a merry-go-around. By the time the ball hits that spot they have already moved on. That's how I remember it," Faye said.

"Yes, that's a lovely analogy, Faye," James complimented.

"I love rainbows, they make me happy," Carmen continued.

"That's because you are expecting to find a pot of gold at its end," James joked.

"When you see a rainbow, the rain is in front of you and the sun is at the back," Fiona said.

"Where's the gold then?" James was not finished.

"At either end. You just have to find one end," Rowan joined in.

"As sound travels slower than light, this information can be used to estimate the distance of an approaching storm by noting the timing between the lightning and thunder to get a rough estimate. Every second later means a three hundred and thirty metres delay. That's useful information sometimes at open air parties," Fiona concluded.

The food had succeeded in detracting the blood circulation somewhat away from the brain towards the digestive areas and aided by the beer imbibition, James was feeling the soporific effect and was soon paying his own sleep debt supinely. His snoring was beginning to confuse the bird calls in the vicinity. The girls and Rowan decided to go on a short hike.

Carmen chose to rest next to James. She was exhausted as she had woken up early to fulfil the meal requirements for the trip and was quite pleased with the results. As always, they had all enjoyed her efforts and just for that, her life was worthwhile. She had come a long way both physically and mentally. Here was James resting just next to her. She remembered him as the much younger man and their Breach Candy exploits in Bombay. She remembered Rowan growing up and her own mother's determination. She must write to Cecil. She wished his family was here as well. But knowing Cecil that would not have been possible. He never liked his comfort zone threatened. Esther was the perfect wife for him. One day maybe his children would come to Australia to visit their cousin, Rowan. She was sure Rowan would marry a local girl. She really had no objections to that. Ultimately our culture must give way here, she thought. If there is no god, what can explain all the mysterious ways? Do I really need an explanation?

She felt sleep creeping on her when she heard the voices of the returning hikers nearby.

James woke up, "Sorry I fell asleep Carmen."

"That's okay" she replied wishing for a nonsexual encounter tonight.

"I think we should go. It is getting a bit cold," Fatima said.

"I agree," Fiona echoed.

They packed their belongings and Rowan drove the Land Rover back.

On the way home the back seat occupants were soon all sleep and James and Rowan decided to aid them by not indulging in any conversation.

On arrival home everyone appeared tired and begged for some light sandwiches only. There would be no discussion tonight. They were grateful to Fatima who had already left for bed much before the others.

Tomorrow they would be ready for a difficult topic if possible, Rowan thought. Please Fatima please will it so!

The others parted with the usual goodnight

choruses.

33

Both Rowan and James were not on call tonight. Every voluntary muscle fibre in Rowan's body was technically eligible for relaxation. Whether the individual fibres were aware of this allowance or not, Rowan was not himself fully informed. In hospital matters his objective was always to be in the prepared mode whether on duty or not. Situations had arisen in the past when local fellow doctors and nurses had taken advantage of his obliging nature. Rowan never complained nor even understood that he was being used and always considered himself as lending a helping hand to his team. Doctors at the JJ Hospital were trained to accept long hours of work as a part of the job of being a doctor.

The waning crescent moon was on its last session tonight before yielding to a new moon tomorrow. The evening air was warm as it moved in preformed routes in the room as dictated by its predecessor flow and as if a prepaid toll on the subject route had to be spent in toto. The warmth was interpreted by James and Rowan as an invitation to wear singlcts and shorts. The ladies contributed the colour and particularly Carmen with her multi flowered kaftan. The family was not yet aware of James' clandestine plan. Everyone was equipped with a glass of wine. Before Fatima could provide the ingredients for the topic tonight she was pre-empted by James, "I would like to suggest the topic for today."

"Okay dad," Rowan replied. He was beginning to accept his position in the family now.

James reciprocated with, "I want to talk a bit about quantum physics today son. Do you know much about it?"

"No. My knowledge about the subject is really tending toward absolute zero," Rowan admitted.

The girls were suddenly thrust with a topic that they had vague plans to deal with individually at some time in the future and were delighted to accept an introduction now. Carmen had wanted to know about it for a long time and what it was all about but was always told it was only for the very brilliant minds. Humbly she had accepted it was not her turf.

"That would be very interesting dad. I want to know," Fiona replied.

"I will listen. I am hoping the wine you poured for me will help," Carmen said.

"Although the mathematics is mind boggling, it is possible to grasp the tenets without the entire math," James said.

"In that case, my wine will really help," Carmen joked.

"In school they teach you classical Newtonian physics which works for the big world but fails completely to explain things in the small world of atoms which actually is the real world," James began.

"Interesting," Faye was all ears. She always wished to take the topic head on one day. And the day had arrived she thought. She wished she had done some little prior reading.

"As long as you remember, it is weird and we have to shed a few of our reality concepts, you will be okay," James warned.

"In India we have no reality. So I might already be good at it James," Carmen joked.

"There are a few Indians who understand it very well Carmen. You may be ahead of me already," James replied.

"Abracadabra," Fiona recited.

"I don't mean magic Fiona. Quantum physics challenges our general logic of location, causality and reality. In the quantum field, these principles actually completely disappear."

"I have always thought so, particularly when you get cranky with me sometimes for no particular reason," Fatima smiled.

"You mean there is nothing to say because of, in quantum physics," Rowan understood.

"Sort of. The physicist, Max Planck in 1899 discovered that energy comes in quanta which is fixed packet amounts rather than a continuous flow," James continued.

"Rather like sugar crystals rather than icing sugar when you pour it out," Fatima said.

"Good analogy Fatima," James complimented her.

"Natural numbers rather than all the rational numbers," Faye added.

"Sort of. Remember if you don't understand anything, that is okay. You are normal. You will understand everything in your own time. As you all know the smallest form of matter is the atom which is made up of particles called protons and neutrons and electrons which are further made up of only two kinds of particles, quarks and leptons. The quarks are the strongly interacting particles that form protons and neutrons. The leptons are the lighter ones, such as the electrons or the neutrinos that come out of the sun. These particles interact with one another through some fairly simple and well-understood forces—the electroweak force, the strong nuclear force, and gravity. How are we going?"

"I think I am normal. I don't understand anything," Carmen admitted.

"I am trying," Fiona said with puzzled look on her face.

"So far so good for me," Faye said.

"I'm okay so far," Rowan replied.

"I am going to go through with this with you but it is best to read it yourself sometime. You will pick it up much better. Do you want me to continue?" James asked.

"Yes, please," Rowan pleaded. He wondered why he had never picked up a book on quantum physics himself in all this while.

"Okay there are a few fundamentals we should get from the beginning. Remember I used the word, weird," James continued.

"Go slow. I want to try to get it right from the beginning," Fatima said.

"All matter is also energy. So we will call it matterenergy here. All matterenergy is in constant motion," James went on.

"Matterenergy sounds like maternity," Carmen said.

"It does, doesn't it? Maybe it has something to do with mother earth," Fiona added.

"Quantum physics is the description of microscopic motion. Such motion is not detected by our senses and therefore we cannot see or feel it. The basic particles besides being matterenergy are also waves and hence they have wave properties too." James continued.

"As energy can be converted into matter and vice versa according to Einstein's famous equation it seems plausible to me to deduce that it can be both a particle and a wave. A sort of duality characteristic," Rowan understood.

"Right," James replied and continued further, "These particles exist in distinct states called quanta."

"That's easy," Rowan said.

"A travelling particle cannot be located until it is actually detected. In other words when travelling from Sydney to Brisbane we cannot say it will be or was in Newcastle at a particular time. Unless of course we look for and catch it in Newcastle. But in doing so we have disrupted its further travel plans."

"So far so good," Fiona mentioned.

"Also in the microdomain, when we conduct an experiment the result is never predictable. The result is always probalistic never definitive," James continued.

Like Jonny Mathis' *Chances are*. Chances are awfully good we may understand this," Rowan joked,

"I like that," Carmen appeared interested.

"Wait till you hear this. Particles can be in superposition. This means that if you can know the properties of a particle A in Newcastle, you can decipher the properties of its superposed partner B holidaying in Hawaii or on the planet Jupiter and even send a message to it. When particles interact with each other in such a way that each is dependent on the other, they are known to be in quantum entanglement. The ability of the individual states of a quantum superposition to interfere with each other is destroyed, or severely degraded, by the environment. Knowledge of the superposition by the outside world is all that is needed to destroy it."

Faye thought she would like to send a message to Freida but soon realised that, that would require supernatural rather than superposition powers.

"A particle travelling from point A to B takes all possible paths to get there. That means to travel from Sydney to Brisbane it would go through Newcastle, Melbourne, Adelaide, Perth, Darwin and all in between routes at the same time," James continued.

"This is really weird dad, as you mentioned," Faye said.

"It is possible only to observe only the consequences of an atom being in two places at once, but not it actually being in two places at once. In other words we can never observe a quantum system directly. We can only observe its effect on its environment," James explained.

Both Carmen and Fatima were beginning to succumb to the soporific effect of the topic. Fatima thought she would read more about it later in her own time and preferred only to listen at this stage. Carmen decided this matter does not matter to her.

"So all matterenergy is both a particle and a wave spreading through space, all reality is only probabilistic which means it is not fixed and may be different depending on chance and all our measurements at an atomic level are uncertain because we interfere with the physical atom to measure it. That is why atoms can be at two places at one time, have spooky connections and can go through barriers which is called tunneling," James summarised

"Weird it is," Rowan interjected.

"However way you want to understand it, its okay. So once again, remember, atoms can be in two or more places at once, penetrate impenetrable barriers, and know about each other instantly even when on different sides of the Universe. They are also totally unpredictable. Every electron is identical to every other electron, every photon is identical to every other photon, and so on. Understood?"

"It sort of makes nonsensical sense," Rowan retorted again.

"If two events in the microscopic world are indistinguishable, the waves associated with them interfere. So a bit about waves will help here now since we are also dealing with waves. Two travelling waves can either help each other and add or destroy each other and subtract in varying amount depending on whether they are in more synchrony or less in synchrony," James continued.

"Like what you see when you throw a pebble in the pond at Blackbutt Reserve and see the tiny wave ripples," Fiona said.

"Yeah I have also done that," Faye joined.

"An electromagnetic wave has two components, electric and magnetic which travel at right angles to each other. Electricity in motion generates magnetism and magnetism in motion generates electricity," James continued. He appeared to be in full swing of his diction now.

"I get it. We did those experiments in school when we moved a magnet and generated a current in a coil of wire," Faye added.

"Imagine electric and magnetic waves travelling at right angles to each other and as they do so, generating more and more magnetic and electric waves, in the whole universe," James continued.

"I can't even think, my brain needs to evolve further," Faye admitted.

Also, have you heard of *Schrödinger's* cat?" James continued.

"Who hasn't? But tell us more about it," Fiona asked.

"Yes. We know about the radioactivity and the poison vial," Faye added.

"You know the idea of the experiment. It is a beautiful effort to demonstrate a micro event with a macro analogy that we all can understand. It demonstrates that until we open the box we do not know whether the cat is alive or dead. In the microworld every atom is in a super position, dead and alive at the same time until we find and localise it, which is similar to opening the box," James continued.

"I understand now," Fiona admitted.

"A sort of we don't know until we locate it,"

Rowan said.

"And when these atoms unite to form larger molecules they get pushed into the macroworld and become objects that we can sense but eventually everything that is observed is affected by the observer," James added.

"So we see things differently," Rowan interpreted.

"Exactly. It means that everyone sees a different truth because everyone is creating what they see," James agreed.

"Wow, you have opened my eyes to a new direction dad. I certainly need to chase this further," Rowan declared.

"Remember, the universe of quantum mechanics and classical physics are different because they explain reality from different points of view. In classical physics, something happens for a purpose. Nothing occurs by accident; it happens because it is caused by something else. In quantum physics however, reality does not occur in terms of reason and effect but on the basis of probability. Nevertheless, the results obtained in quantum physics are very accurate," James added.

Carmen looked at James in amazement. She thought how do you know so much? And you are mine now. How can it be?

"I'll bet there must be a lot more to know," Fiona admitted.

"Yes much more. All electromagnetic waves travel at the speed of light. Light itself is also an electromagnetic wave. If matterenergy was ever to attain the speed of light itself, it would acquire an infinite mass, and moving it would take an infinite amount of energy which is not available in the entire Universe. So this is an impossibility. Time stops at the speed of light. So this can't ever happen. Only photons which are light particles and are massless can move at the speed of light," James could see that this was getting too weighty for his listeners and thought it best to leave them to explore further in their own time. He had laid the foundations as he had planned.

Then as a parting shot, "Quantum physics, arguably is the greatest triumph of human intelligence and imagination in all of history. According to quantum physics, what we can observe about the world is only a tiny subset of what actually exists. Read it yourself but don't give up. Eventually it will click and you will get your mind around it," James finished.

"Yes we'll read some more and we must discuss it again another time. It is very interesting," Faye added.

Fatima looked confused. She knew she had a lot of catching up to do.

"That was certainly most interesting dad. I think in medicine the psychiatrists could derive a lot of benefit from this knowledge," Rowan worked out.

"Yes, I agree with you Rowan particularly in the psychoses," Carmen added. She had been listening and had picked up the fundamentals. She had also decided to chase the subject further herself.

"Mostly medicine only needs classical Newtonian mechanics. But in the psychoses realm, reality as we know it in the big world is disturbed and the schizophrenic minds may be using a quantum plane to interpret their reality. Some autistic minds like the *Rain Man* may also function at this level," Rowan theorised.

"That's a very interesting observation, Rowan. I never thought it that way. I wonder if the psychiatrists would see it that way," James admitted.

"Also it occurred to me that if atoms can tunnel through, it is possible that evolution has employed this trick to use the same neurotransmitter to perform different functions as required by the Schrödinger moment. For example dopamine is responsible for several functions like pleasure, physical movement, motivation, learning etcetera, all different functions. A single atom of the same molecule of dopamine could tunnel and occupy different positions at separate times to fulfil the different needs. If nature can do this it is substance economy for functional utility at its best. Isn't it? The same cloth being used as a dress, a table cloth and bed sheet. The exact temporal effect may be determined by the Schrödinger's cat effect at that particular time. Like if you are in the bedroom, dining room or the dressing room," Rowan continued.

James himself was overwhelmed. He had produced his own quantum Frankenstein right here! He wanted time to think that one out. But it appeared almost feasible. He was very proud of Rowan. Perhaps they could both have quantrums – quantum tantrums with the girls?

There was silence in the room with everyone lost in

thought. Fatima resolved that she would catch up. The subject is fascinating. She had books to find. James would help. Faye would read more and see if it was possible to communicate with the supernatural with quantum physics. Who knows? There may be a way. Fiona was undecided whether she should take the maths on as she was quite good at mathematics at school particularly at calculus. It would be a massive effort. No. she won't, she decided. Rowan thought he could explore the quantum features of the disturbed human mind with help from Carmen when suddenly a human voice brought them all back, "Now to the macroworld for some real food for thought and that reminds me I have to pick up some butter and eggs tomorrow," Carmen reminded herself loudly.

They were all exhausted with this weird thinking exercise and a large quantum of sleep would be most welcome. With those thoughts in mind they parted for the night.

Consciousness was soon lost by all except James who pondered if he could have made the topic any easier especially for Carmen. But not now. She was fast asleep.

34

It was obvious that the united semirelated families would get along quite well. They all had similar characteristics, curiosity for knowledge and the desire to share it and a unabating fascination with Indian food. None of the members of this family indulged in small talk. James had learnt that from his own upbringing. Rodney and Elena never encouraged small talk. He had always felt that happiness and purpose could only be found in perpetual curiosity.

He knew he was finally really home. Home geographically, home professionally, home romantically and home with his offspring. Freida did haunt his sentimental memory at times but reality usually won. Carmen was a perfect wife and Rowan and the girls left nothing to be desired nor did they invade his own comfort boundaries, but as always in life there is always one more problem left to deal with. Fiona and Faye needed to find reliable husbands.

In the matter of Fiona there may be an opening. A co-physiotherapist christened John Kennedy whom James and Carmen had both met was working in the same department with Fiona. He was demanding Fiona's romantic attention. He was a tall photogenic redhead with an athletic build that seemed to convince his clients that perhaps he knew what he was doing. Fiona often spent her evenings in his company.

John's father was of Irish descent and his mother was English and John was always critical of their obsessions, his father being a perfectionist and his mother having an obsessive fear of contamination and dirt. John mentioned how as a child his mother always insisted on cleaning the bench they would sit on in the park with Dettol wipes. His mother often spent her entire day at home just cleaning. His father was an accountant who spent his time, not trusting the computer calculations and rechecked the calculations himself several times to detect if there were any errors in his own calculations. Partly as a result, his father was late home in the evenings and early back to work next morning. John himself considered parents were the bane of society. He had worked that out from school. He remembered how his packed school lunches always comprised of fruit and cooked vegetables while all the other school children delighted their taste buds with the oil baptised pastries from the canteen. What a wonderful world this would be if there were just no parents!

John expected Fiona's sympathy for his perceived woes and Fiona mostly obliged by providing the obligatory listen and concerned look. Fiona knew how lucky she was with her own parents. At times she tried to convince him that his current physique may be related to his mother's diet and his own school colleagues may be now challenging the restrictions imposed by the extra very large sizes at the clothes stores. However John was not convinced and always talked about a neglected and missed childhood. But he was a good lover.

Twinges of a hibernating Irish accent, at times contaminated by Hackney cockney overtones betrayed his dual lineage. Fiona also loved to hear him speak which really turned her on. John boasted that his grandparents lived next door to Jessica Tandy before she moved to the US as if such credentials should be considered in a marital deal. Who was Jessica Tandy? Fiona wondered but preferred not to ask or want to know.

Faye was still opaque in her personal inclinations and preferred to be secretive. She had thought about her future but was not in a hurry to be involved in a romantic encounter yet. Some male hopefuls had expressed their desire to associate with her but she had politely declined. She often thought about Freida. Why did she have to go? Could there be anything she herself could have done that could have helped? Not that she did not like Carmen. She adored both Carmen and Rowan. Eventually what has to happen will happen.

Fatima was on her gap year and scheduled to go to Sydney University to study medicine soon. She spent her time mostly reading books on quantum physics and often involving James and Rowan in a quantrum.

Carmen accepted her lot and good luck. She was happy that Rowan had finally found his father and she, her much longed and now loved husband. She was happy that Rowan was James' son in spite of all the humiliation she had endured in Byculla along with her mother and Cecil in those days. She remembered the days, how when she had attempted to walk down the street when pregnant with Rowan in Byculla, how the young children would often follow her chanting, "Hail Carmen, full of grapes" possibly coached by their satanic parents. How she had felt like catching each one of them and disjointing them, one bone at a time and enjoying their cries of pain. Her own mental pain at that time was all worth it now. Her mother Felicity would forgive her for everything now. It is amazing how the individual human mind can forget and forgive any misery provided the outcome is ultimately beneficial to all concerned. She only wished her own mother, was here to enjoy her good luck!

Rowan appeared to be finally at peace with himself. As a child he had always felt sad that he never got to meet his father. Looking back he understood why there were no photos of his dad at Byculla. He always felt that being a plastic surgeon would help him get closer to his dead father's memory but in fact it did so in a live father! What a bonus!

James had plans for Rowan which he hoped to spell out soon.

One Thursday evening when the family was gathered for their postprandial discourses, James inquired, "Rowan, have you decided on your future plans here?"

"No, not yet. You will have to guide me on that."

"I think you should be eligible to sit the part two of the Fellowship exam which is a written and viva.

You should write to the Australasian College of Surgeons promptly and get your eligibility confirmed and then sit the exam."

"Indeed, I shall do that tomorrow."

"And after you pass then you can join me in my rooms."

"Wow. I so look forward to that."

"Remember the fellowship is a very difficult exam. Not that the exam itself is difficult but somehow the failure rate is very high."

"Why is that?" Rowan was intrigued.

"Possibly because the marking is done by humans who are subject to some bias," James explained.

"That problem is universal. In India, it is the nepotism clock that remains ticking when acquiring any qualification or employment."

"We just have to deal with that in life. By the way, Carmen, I have to call the plumber in tomorrow. The shower is leaking a bit."

"I suppose we will get another fat invoice," Carmen was not happy.

"Plumbers also have bills to pay. Live and let live"

At this moment the silence was suddenly interrupted by Fatima who wanted to know,

"Dad are you going to have any more kids?"

James smiled at Carmen and Carmen reciprocated.

A thought went through Carmen's mind. Indeed 'God works in mysterious ways'. And another in James' mind 'The outcomes in quantum physics are unpredictable'.

Unbeknown to all, Rowan had been secretly dating Imogen, a quantum physicist lecturer at the

University. She was the sister of Fatima's friend, Natalie whom they had visited about a month before to watch the finches, at their father's aviary in Wallsend.

Rowan could remember the exact moment when Imogen Carden entered the aviary and how he was completely speechless on seeing her. She was about five feet and five inches tall with hazel eyes and dark brown shoulder length hair. Something was also happening to him in his genital regions and his dial was rising to indicate a 'full tank'. This was indeed love and love at first sight he thought. He was never allowed to think this can happen.

"Hi Imogen, this is Rowan, Fatima's brother," Natalie introduced him.

"Fatima, you never told me that you had a brother," Imogen looked puzzled.

"You never asked me," Fatima's replied.

Imogen could not take her eyes off Rowan. She attempted to explain finch behaviour to him herself and slowly led him away from Fatima and Natalie and requested his contact details. Rowan tongue rolled her request. She was fascinated by his accent. His tongue roll did not bother her. She had heard from Natasha about James' tongue rolling speech. Obviously a family trait, she thought. If things did get serious she could live with it. But how could she explain his accent? She would have time now to find that out.

They dated a few times, often for an evening meal and Rowan usually arriving late, armed with pardonable excuses which Imogen felt she could live with. She just loved being with him and he with her.

After their meal this particular evening, they decided to go for a walk. Imogen found a deserted bench on which they parked themselves. Imogen longed to kiss him. She had waited long enough.

"Rowan, will you please kiss me tonight?"

"I'm very sorry Imogen, I don't know how to kiss. If you can teach me, I can try."

"I'd love to," and she put her arms around his neck

Rowan remembered the western movies he had seen in India. He put his hands round her waist and pulled her close. The mouths locked. And so the lesson began with Rowan conscious of his tongue rolling and whether it would interfere with his performance. Both the teacher and student enjoyed the initial experience. As usual, Rowan wanted to perfect his technique and asked for more trials and Imogen was more than happy to oblige. She was catching up for all the times she had missed before. Imogen could feel his genital anatomy going on full alert. She was feeling her own nipples tighten and her pelvic regions were beginning to respond. Suddenly Rowan decided to stop, for fear of complications that he may not know how to handle. Less is more he thought, as he was taught in plastic surgery and pulled away.

At this exact moment the mouths parted and the tongues retracted into their home territories. They separated and both of them burst out laughing. A hurdle had been overcome and things would move faster now. They parted with another prolonged kiss and with arrangements when to meet next. At least kissing would be easier now!

But for Rowan there was another major hurdle. Carmen had warned him several times about marrying a local girl and he was aware that uncle Cecil was on a mission to find him the gastroenterologist wife in Byculla. He could never disappoint Carmen. No matter what. He would rather die. Should he stop Imogen before things get out of control? Who could advise him in this matter? James? But he would let Carmen know. Should he take it head on with Carmen? No. Just watching the look on her face would kill him. After all she had been through for him! She could have had an abortion with him. She chose not to. She had given him his life and more. He could never and will ever, disappoint her. To his surprise, suddenly he had an answer.

He would consult Rodney and Elena. They are always nice to him. Surely he could talk to them in confidence. They would understand and they could intervene on his behalf with Carmen who held them both in very high regard.

Oftentimes when he was not on duty, Rowan had visited Rodney and Elena at their vineyard. They had let him know that they loved having him over. Rodney and Elena both admired him and Carmen, and often wondered about the hardships they might have been through in their own Indian culture, as a result of their son, James. They never spared James their thoughts whenever they could. As a result, James was beginning to despise visiting them and restricted his visits only to the ultra-festive occasions.

Rowan rang Elena and asked if he could visit on the coming Saturday.

'Of course you are most welcome Rowan."

He did not inform anyone at home and went to see Elena and Rodney.

At the vineyard, both Rodney and Elena fussed greatly over him.

"What brings you here today Rowan?" Elena asked.

"Yes. Tell us," Rodney also wanted to know.

"I have a problem," and Rowan went on to explain as they both listened intently. Rodney and Elena both remembered their own similar problems. Rodney's parents were not keen on Elena.

"I will talk to Carmen," Elena volunteered.

"Yes, its best that you do it. Only women can understand women," Rodney said.

"It is important that you are not there Rowan," Elena said.

"I can easily arrange not to be there."

On his way home Rowan thought he may be jumping the gun. He had been carried away by his emotions. He had not talked about marriage with Imogen. But under the current circumstances he really couldn't. He was intending to ask Imogen to marry him only if Elena was successful in convincing Carmen. And if Elena was, only then he would ask Imogen to marry him. He saw very little hope. Nevertheless some ground may still be gained in the long run.

Elena arranged with Carmen to meet for coffee in

the city. Rodney would drive her in and find his way to the Angus and Robertson bookshop nearby whilst Elena would inveigle Carmen into her eugenic assignment from Rowan.

Carmen was pleased with the invitation and really did not want to analyse any motives as an Indian mind usually would, and not definitely with Elena and Rodney. She trusted them totally.

On being informed about Rowan's plight by Elena, Carmen responded, "I have thought about that Elena, and I really hoped that something like that would happen. I am pleased to hear what you have told me. I will speak to Rowan myself tonight"

Having discussed the exact plotting with Rodney the night before and having rehearsed all the answers and possible objections from Carmen, Elena found her task with Carmen went very well. They could now enjoy their coffee. And Rowan would be grateful.

That evening when Rowan was back home from work, he was summoned by Carmen to her bedroom and her position on the matter was spelled out to him.

"Do you have anyone in mind?" Carmen asked.

"No. Not yet, but I just wanted to keep the coast clear," Rowan lied.

"Okay. That's good. I am so proud of you."

"Thank you mum"

That evening Rowan was due for a dinner date with Imogen. He would definitely be on time on this occasion. After their last encounter, he felt he may not be able to hold on with his sexual urges for long. She had started him on a different path, a road he had not trodden on before. He was thinking and dreaming about her most of the time now. He wondered if he should ask her to marry him tonight. Then she could be with him for most of his nonworking hours. He would be almost independent soon and James had assured him of a job on passing the Fellowship exam for which he had already applied for. Carmen was attended to and was happy. So why not?

And so it came to pass, "Imogen, will you marry me?" he asked her.

"Really Rowan, we hardly know each other that well to think of getting married. Don't you think?"

Rowan did not expect this answer.

Getting to know each other that well? That well before marriage? Don't you think we know enough about each other already? What we know about each other so far is a lot more than I expected. Rowan did not comprehend.

He had a lot more to learn.

UNDOING BANDAGES: A PLASTIC NOVEL

It's always a nice feeling to know that you've affected someone's life, maybe changed it a bit or just gave them a reminder of a thing that they've already known.

Thank you

A b o u t   t h e   A u t h o r

The author is a semiretired ear nose throat and facial cosmetic surgeon with a legal degree and now does medicolegal work mainly. He has written papers for international refereed journals on ear and sinus surgery and provided a new theory for tinnitus causation, based on evolutionary principles. He has also provided a novel technique for ear membrane grafting. Writing a self published novel was an experience, particularly to learn everything from editing to formatting! As a result, I will reserve the right to maintain ownership of all the errors.

www.svfernandes.com

Acknowledgments

First and foremost I wish to thank my wife Celine and my children, Meyrelle, Keyoren, Kersten and Ryelen who at various times have lightened my burden by providing disposable and indisposable comments. My thanks also go to Dr. Barney D'Costa who provided beta reader help.

UNDOING BANDAGES: A PLASTIC NOVEL